THE ANDERSON METHOD®

The Secret
to Permanent Weight Loss

By William Anderson, MA, LMHC
Forward by Mark Lupo, MD

www.TheAndersonMethod.com

Two Harbors Press
212 3rd Avenue North, Suite 570
Minneapolis, MN 55401
612.455.2293
www.TwoHarborsPress.com

ISBN - 978-1-935097-28-0
ISBN - 1-935097-28-8
LCCN - 2008911001

Book sales for North America and international:
Itasca Books, 3501 Highway 100 South, Suite 220
Minneapolis, MN 55416
Phone: 952.345.4488 (toll free 1.800.901.3480)
Fax: 952.920.0541; email to orders@itascabooks.com

Cover Design by Meghan Gale
Typeset by James Arneson

Printed in the United States of America

THE ANDERSON METHOD®

The Secret
to Permanent Weight Loss

*Dedicated to my
Clients, Patients, and Readers.*

CONTENTS

FOREWORD

Read This First
By Mark Lupo M.D.

When my first patient came back one hundred pounds lighter, healthier and happier, after following The Anderson Method, it got my attention. She tried to get a handle on her weight problem for years. When we first met, she thought reaching her ideal weight was impossible. She felt hopeless. She was suffering from diabetes and high blood pressure. She hated her body, and her weight was getting worse.

I had just learned of psychotherapist Bill Anderson's unique weight control method, and she was the first patient I referred to it. Imagine my surprise when she appeared for her next visit having lost fifty pounds! And she said it was easy! Then she came back having lost one hundred pounds. Now at 120 pounds at five feet, four inches, her success is something none of us could have imagined.

And that was just the beginning. Patient after patient started returning for follow-up visits after being referred to The Anderson Method. They all had similar stories. They were solving their "impossible" weight problems, shedding the extra pounds and the health and emotional problems that came with them, and calling it "easy." I knew something very new and very big was happening.

I am an Endocrinologist, a doctor who specializes in metabolic disorders and the endocrine system, the body's network of glands that send the chemical messengers that are the language of your physiology. I trained with the country's top experts in medical weight loss, the doctors who most want to find a medical solution to our number one preventable public health hazard—obesity. When patients seemed to stay overweight no matter what they did, doctors sent them to me for treatment with pharmacologic therapies and clinical dietitians.

It was supposed to be a straight-forward process. The problem was, most of these patients didn't have glandular problems. The mystery was many of them didn't seem to eat any differently than thin people, yet still had excessive weight gain. After working together for a while, we found that the problem was more of a lifestyle problem than a metabolic one. They just couldn't live with what they had to do to lose weight and couldn't live without doing things that made them gain weight. Their habits had control of them, and they felt helplessly in the grip of their food addictions. Medication and surgery couldn't address their underlying problems. Even if the patients lost weight with a "quick fix," it didn't change their lifestyles, and they gained the weight back. We didn't have a way for patients to get control of the habits and compulsions that had control of them.

In April of 2004, I met psychotherapist Bill Anderson. He intrigued me with his behavioral program of Therapeutic Psychogenics and his own success over his severe weight problem. The program's objective, he explained, was to create a permanent change in habitual behavior and thinking. I knew from my experience with patients, and medical research, that a comprehensive behavioral approach like his was the answer.

He explained most clients' problems as akin to addiction. Bells went off in my head. I knew he was on the right track, and I started referring patients to him to see if he could help.

The rest, as they say, is history. Scores of patients started coming back with their success stories. They lost significant amounts of weight and achieved greater success than medications produced. They were able to stop taking medications for high blood pressure and diabetes. They had more energy and less depression. The very same patients who six months earlier had hoped a thyroid problem would be the explanation for their "inability" to lose weight were back, happy to have finally found a solution that worked. As more learned of the results his methods produced, his waiting list grew to more than a year to be able to see him. He has now trained associates in his method to duplicate his success.

Now he has written this book to introduce his ideas to you. Linda Carson, the ABC7 news anchor, lost seventy pounds and her lifetime weight problem with The Anderson Method. She and I think that just reading this book can enable a person to solve their weight problem. Perhaps you can find the answer to your weight problem in these pages. However, don't try to be your own doctor, especially if you have conditions like high blood pressure or diabetes. If you decide to make changes so you can lose weight, check with your doctor to make sure you're still doing what you need to do to be healthy.

Whether you need to engage in a formal program or not, the seeds to your success are in the following pages. Through learning about The Anderson Method, I have come to believe that success is possible, no matter how much you have struggled and failed. This book will put you on the right track, in a world where it has been terribly obscured.

I have devoted my life to the healing arts. There have been so many times I have wished to change things that were just beyond my ability to control. So, I am so happy to be able

CHAPTER 1

Addicted

We are a nation of addicts, a world of addicts. We seem helplessly caught in our addiction to consuming, consuming ourselves to death.

We are eating ourselves sick, becoming fatter and fatter every year, while knowing that our obesity and our obesity epidemic are becoming the greatest threats to our health and our healthcare system. We are unable to stop it. We define ourselves not as citizens, or neighbors, or even people, but as "consumers."

As good consumers, we overeat. We consume too much; that's why we are overweight and obese.

Before you read any further, let's get one thing straight. You have a weight problem because you overeat. You habitually eat more food than you need. If you are in the habit of pretending that you really don't eat too much, that the problem is because of something else, as if you'd stay overweight even if you ate very little, you need to stop it. People who don't eat a lot get thin. If they eat next to nothing, they will eventually waste away and die. There were no fat people in the famines of Biafra or

Ethiopia, or in Nazi Germany's Auschwitz. You are in the habit of overeating, eating more than you need, and it has made you chronically overweight. You have become a good consumer in a culture of consuming. We are the "consumers."

We are consuming the world's resources at record speed, while knowing that it is destroying us, destroying the earth that we depend upon. Our eating habits are ruining us, creating lethal diseases like heart disease and diabetes and robbing us of the ability to fully enjoy our bodies and our lives. Our destruction of the forests and incineration of the oil within the earth is fouling the atmosphere and seas and flooding the continents so that our homes will become unlivable, with nowhere else to go. Our voracious appetites call the shots, leading us to deny the reality that is so obvious: We have been destroying ourselves, consuming ourselves to death.

Like an alcoholic with cirrhosis of the liver, we have pretended that the way we are living is OK, that giving up our lifestyle is an unreasonable and unnecessary sacrifice, and that we can get away with it. We can't.

But, we *can* change. You *can* solve your weight problem. You *can* become the weight you'd like to be. You can learn to enjoy life and eating in a new and better way. You don't have to give up good food or enjoying the good life. You can change for the better. You can lose your excess weight and your weight problem. And as you change yourself, everything changes. You get better, and the world gets better.

Do you want a better life, a better world? Let's start here. Let's solve our obesity problem.

CHAPTER 2

What Is the Problem

You probably think that the problem is your weight. Your clothes are tight. You hate the way you look. You swear you'll be good every morning with a new start, but then you weaken and blow it, and you get mad at yourself, maybe even hate yourself.

You refuse to buy new clothes in a larger size, and you hate the idea of going to the store and finding out what size you are now. You hate it that you have all these clothes that don't fit. You hate thinking that if you had gotten your act together last year, you'd be at your target weight today, and you hate thinking that it will be a year before you'll be happy, even if you started today.

You're afraid to get on the scale and find out what it says. You avoid going to the doctor; you remember the first thing they do is weigh you.

You hate it when people intrude and say things like "I'm just concerned about you." They act like they think you don't realize you have a weight problem or that you don't care, as if overweight people wanted or chose to be fat.

You've dieted, sometimes successfully, but then you've gained it all back and more. It seems like when you eat normally, you gain, as if the only way you could possibly not be fat is to deny yourself real food forever, never again relax and just eat normally. And that is a terrifying and hateful thought. To never again be able to eat in a satisfying way when you get home? Never again go to restaurants the way you like? Vacation the way you like? Have the holidays, dinners, and desserts you like? It's hideous. It's unthinkable. It speaks of a cold life not worth living. And when you contemplate what you've just thought, that's as frightening as anything else you've thought. Has eating become what you live for, the purpose of your life? What have you become?

So, you vow to change, to be good. You want to be different. Your body hurts. You hate the stretch marks. You hate the way the fat bulges out, and you try to hide it. You hate what it does to your shoes and clothes. You hate the threat of high blood pressure, heart disease, heart attack, and diabetes. You hate the pills and the doctor's warnings.

You vow to change, and you join the health club and start the diet. You even convince yourself for a few days that it will work. But then you quit, and you go back to what you know is ruining your life, killing you, and you let it continue killing you. What will become of you? What have you become?

You have become an addict. And unless you beat it, it will rob you of the great life you can have. It will ruin everything.

CHAPTER 3

It's Not Just *Your* Problem

Of course, you are not the only one with this problem. In fact, it is now normal to be very overweight.

Today, two-thirds of the adults in America are clinically overweight. What's "clinically overweight?" A woman who is five feet, four inches is clinically overweight if she weighs 145 pounds…

One-third of us is *clinically obese*. That would be 174 for our five foot, four inch woman. A man six feet tall would be obese at 221.

Now, if something in you right now wants to deny this, wants to say that 145 or 221 aren't that bad… that's the addict talking, like the guy with cirrhosis of the liver saying he's got a "little" cirrhosis, "not that bad."

Obese is an ugly word. I've always hated it. Rhymes with grease. Most people are shocked when they see it in their medical chart or hear the doctor use it to describe them. They knew they weighed too much, but until they faced the word "obese," they were able to think that they were "big boned," or "hefty," or "husky." When the doctors apply the label *obese*, it sounds serious, and it is. Obese is sick.

One-third of us are obese, *one-third*, <u>sick</u>, because of our overeating. It wasn't always this way. When did this happen?

~

In 1976 to 1980, about fifteen percent of us were obese. So we've *doubled* the rate in the *last thirty years*. The obesity rate in kids has *quadrupled* in that same period. If we are not able to get a handle on this problem, where will we be in thirty years? Will two-thirds of us be obese? Three-quarters?

And you only have to look to your own experience with your eating habits and weight to wonder how difficult or easy it will be to reverse this trend. Threatening, isn't it?

In the 70's, the U.S. Surgeon General linked smoking to cancer and declared war, and more than twenty percent of us still smoke! What do you think is going to happen with overeating? Smoking is an easy habit to break compared to overeating. Can you imagine what will happen in this country if two-thirds or three-quarters of us are obese? The obesity trend will make smoking seem insignificant as a health issue.

Our government's Center for Disease Control and Prevention, the "CDC" that you hear about with AIDS, HIV, and SARS, has declared obesity an "epidemic." *An epidemic!* Right now, it is the second leading cause of preventable death in the country, and it will probably overtake smoking in the next several years. That's only taking into account the early deaths that obesity causes and not looking at the suffering and expense of all the non-fatal illness it causes. What's worse, the epidemic is just beginning.

Obesity is increasing at rates that in the past were only seen with infectious diseases. It's spreading like a plague. It's worse than smoking. It has the potential to overwhelm our health care system and our economy.

Obesity is known to dramatically increase (500 percent in some cases) the risks for diabetes, heart disease, high blood pressure, cancers, and disability. It's not just hateful and miserable for the individual to be overweight. As a nation, it threatens to break the health care system and bankrupt us. According to the 2001 Surgeon General's Call to Action to Prevent and Decrease Overweight and Obesity, the cost to us nationally that year, due to overweight and obesity was *$117 billion*. I wonder what it is now and what it will be in another thirty years?

No matter how we organize our health care system, we can never produce enough health care to match the disease we can create with our addictions out of control, with this epidemic growing wildly as it is. It's like trying to bail out a sinking ship without plugging the leaks, with the leaks getting bigger. It's senseless to concentrate only on the bailing, even if we do a heroic job. Even with the best bailing, the ship will sink if the leaks continue. If the epidemic trend continues, we will be sunk.

No, you are not alone with this problem, and, no, we're not destined to sink. You are reading this book, and that means you will learn what needs to be done to solve your own weight problem. To stop the epidemic, to save the world, you need to focus on your own solution, and that will change everything. Changing yourself will change everything in you and around you.

We have been afflicted with a plague, but when you get better, it can spread in the same way, like a wound miraculously healing. *You* are the solution to our epidemic and our healthcare crisis.

If we keep going the way we have been, we will suffer a miserable fate. But we can change. Change yourself, and you'll change the world.

CHAPTER 4

Losing the Weight
and Getting Better.

You may be able to take what you learn from this book and solve your weight problem yourself, without engaging in the program of therapy I developed. If so, that will be absolutely wonderful. One of my greatest dreams will have been realized—to be able to write a book that will so enhance a person's life.

But if you find you need help, don't think that you are a failure because you can't do it on your own after reading this book. Everyone is different, with different needs and circumstances. What you learn from this book will help you to get better, regardless of your individual needs and circumstances. It will bring you closer to what you seek, and what you learn here will never be lost. You will never be the same. You will be better.

I got better, and so can you.

When I finally "got it," I lost 140 pounds. I had been overweight my whole life, obese for some time, too. In 1983, I was in my early thirties, and I had been trying to control my weight for the better part of twenty-five years. I was "chunky" or "husky" as a kid, always trying to "watch my weight," and, over time, on every diet on the market. I only got worse as time went by. When I was in my late twenties, I found myself over 300 pounds, with all the miserable thoughts, feelings, and experiences that I shared with you a few pages back.

I'll spare you the soap opera of my whole ordeal, the drama you probably know first hand, and lead you directly to my recovery.

My recovery actually started when I was seven, when I was introduced to my first diet, even though dieting made me more of an overeater than I was before. I tried, and I failed, but I learned. And you have, too.

Over the next twenty-five years, being overweight, dieting, failing, and all the agonies of it, became the central experiences of my life. But in my twenty-five years of failure, I could not help but having learned, and I reached a tipping point of critical mass (excuse the awkward metaphor), and it all came together in my early thirties. I finally "got it."

Coincidently, in those years, I had been moving forward professionally in training people in technique for enhancement of personal achievement. That evolved into work in habit-management training, addictions, and, finally, psychotherapy. The serendipitous coincidence of my personal experience and my professional training seemed to lead me to a unique awareness. I gained insights and knowledge that I think are unavailable to people without this unique "education." I not only "got it" and solved my own weight problem, but I gained the ability to help others.

That serendipitous coincidence, or providential occurrence, however you frame it, was more than twenty years ago now. After twenty-five years of being miserably overweight, I lost 140 pounds, and I have maintained my "Ideal Body Weight," (something I never thought possible, or even wanted) within a few pounds, for more than twenty years.

I'm a licensed psychotherapist now, and I've helped many others to duplicate my success with a remarkably successful approach I call "The Anderson Method." I'm now training other therapists to conduct my method, and my dream is that there will be many therapists all over who can lead people through this process.

Allow me to tell you some of the most important things I learned in my recovery and the development of this approach. Reading this book will not be the same as the experiential learning that occurs in therapy, but, for some, it will be enough to reach their "critical mass," the tipping point to push them into a great success in solving their weight problem. For some, it will be a big step toward their recovery that will lead them to it. Either way, you will learn something vital. You will get better.

CHAPTER 5

Will Power

"You just have to make up your mind," I was told. That was a big lie.

It was a big lie told to me by other people who were just as lost as I was. The difference was, I knew I was lost, and they didn't.

"You have to use will power," I was told, as if it was something I should know how to do. As if it was something everyone knew how to do. As if it was simple. It's not.

When you know you are lost, you look for the way. That's why you're reading this book. When you think you know it all, you talk as if you have all the answers. No doubt, you've run into a few of those, some with credentials and some without. Watch out for those people who act like they have all the answers.

I certainly don't have all the answers— some, but not all.

It's not as simple as "just making up your mind." It's more complex.

They told me to "just use will power," but they could never tell me how, because they didn't know how. Now, I know how.

What I now teach gives people who never had discipline the will power and self control to do things they never thought possible. It has made me into someone who is seen as a person with an iron will, strong discipline, and steely perseverance. *If they only knew.* That image was as far from reality as one could get.

I was named "William." It's ironic. "Will I am." But I was not.

I was probably the biggest example of lack of "will power" that you've ever seen. From the time I was seven into my early thirties, I "just made up my mind" to change, to control myself, to not be fat, *millions* of times, and it didn't work, *millions* of times. Each time I failed, I felt that I was so bad, so weak, so defective. How could anyone be such a failure as to fail at something so simple as "*just* making up your mind?"

I have learned it's *not* just a matter of making up your mind. Having "will power" is not as simple as just making a decision. There are other powers at work. It's complex— and succeeding is a matter of gaining a greater understanding of these powers and learning how to put them to work to be able to make the changes you need, instead of just wishing for them.

You may have the will, the desire and intention, to do what it takes to control your weight, but there are greater powers more often in charge, for most of us. How many times have we prayed and sworn to not eat this or that, or to start doing this or that, experiencing the *immeasurable* heart wrenching desire of one who would give *anything* to lose this weight? Countless times.

Yet, something wells up inside us, with a will of its own, an overpowering force that will have *its* way, to eat something, and then maybe something else, regardless of what *you* want in your most heartfelt dreams and prayers.

How do we overpower it? How does a person who had no will power develop it?

The Anderson Method is an intensive therapeutic program that trains a person to use techniques to do just that and to manage their weight. While a book cannot duplicate what happens in that experience, or include all the science that is learned and employed, it can point the way. This book will acquaint you with some of the powers that drive us, that have made us what we are, that we can use to remake ourselves in a new way.

Each chapter is a piece of the puzzle that will lead to a solution. You already have some. You may have enough when you've finished this book. You may need more. Sit back, and take it in, and see what happens.

CHAPTER 6

Conditioning and Addiction

It's very difficult to easily describe what my method is. In the profession, we use a lot of psychotherapeutic jargon that few understand: behavior therapy; cognitive behavior therapy; cybernetic self-management; psychoeducation; psychotherapeutic eclecticism.

Clients often explain it as "brainwashing." They tell their friends "I'm learning to brainwash myself." That may be the best description.

Some of the most powerful dynamics related to our behavior, our habits, and our toughest habits, our addictions, can be understood as the forces that are recognized in behavioral psychology related to conditioning.

Behaviorists have a rather mechanistic view of human behavior; some seem to deny the existence of free will or consciousness. They are the scientists who see us as white lab rats pushing levers to get food pellets or to stop getting shocked. They see behavior and habits almost as "programs," as if we were computers, the brain being the "hardware." To them, the way we act and think is the software, the "programs."

In their view, the way we act is not a matter of will, but of the programs we have (our habits of thought and action). In their world, the way we act is not a result of will, but of "conditioning." We install or delete programs (habits) according to the principles of *conditioning*, as reliable as what you do with your computer when you download or delete a program.

The cardinal law of behaviorism is: A behavior that is reinforced **will be repeated.** Reinforcement is a matter of having pleasure as a result of the behavior, or at the time of the behavior.

They are saying that if we do something, and it feels good, a power will be created to drive us to do it again. Read that sentence again, just to make sure it sinks in. IF SOMETHING FEELS GOOD, A POWER WILL BE CREATED TO *DRIVE* US TO DO IT AGAIN.

You may say, "well, of course." What could be more obvious? We want to do what feels good.

But I am talking about a power much greater than just liking something.

There is energy at the center of your being, that drives your life, that is much more powerful than your will, and this energy is what the conditioning taps. It is the wellspring of desire, impulse, compulsion, urges, and craving.

You have instinctual drives that will absolutely overpower anything that you "simply" will. These powerful drives come into play automatically, regardless of what you want, and operate on their own, even if you were asleep. The sex drive, for instance, is not something we decide on. It happens to us, sometimes unbidden, and will have its way sometimes, even against our better judgment. Instincts, desire, impulses, compulsion, urges, and craving are drives of this energy, where a baby is driven to suck, a person who is struck, driven to strike back. It is not of the will. It is of another power. It is a power beyond reason, beyond you, the kind of power that fuels survival behavior, maternal behavior, and rivalry.

Conditioning taps into this primal power source, greater than your will, and drives you to repeat behavior that feels good, even if you wanted to stop. Getting the picture?

Many of the addictions can be understood in this context—as "habits on steroids." Cocaine, nicotine, and heroin (some think maybe sugar and chocolate, too) all produce an intense rush of deep pleasure, and your brain knows exactly what to do when something feels that good. Soon, where someone had no interest in drugs, no drive to "use" before getting "hooked," you have an addict who will do anything for the next fix, often things that totally violate their sense of self, their soul, their will.

PLEASURE AND PAIN

Behaviorism ascribes to principles involving pain as well as pleasure.

We will be driven, by that same immense power at our center, to stop things that are painful, to avoid things that are painful, and to do things that stop the pain. We are repelled. Those drug addictions I referred to not only draw the power from the intense pleasure of the fix, but also from the pain of withdrawal. We are driven by repulsion, as well as desire and craving. When addicts start to experience withdrawal, they will begin to be affected by a drive that reaches from a place much deeper than their will. They will seek their fix with the ferocious drive of a drowning swimmer clawing for air.

While some question the existence of a spiritual Higher Power, like God, any addict who has tried to use their will power to stop does not doubt the higher power of their addiction. After countless episodes of swearing you wouldn't do it, praying, promising, using all the will you could summon, and then breaking… you should have no doubt of the power of pleasure and pain and conditioning, of craving, of repulsion. It's not that you had no will power. Something else was bigger.

~

Now, with The Anderson Method, we put this power to work for us, instead of against us. We set up the mechanisms to make us desire and crave what makes us fit and feel repelled by what makes us fat. We use behavior therapy and forms of cognitive behavior therapy, otherwise known as conditioning, or brainwashing. We use our "will power" to decide to engage in the therapy and line up the powers of habit, addiction, craving, and repulsion to serve our will instead of vexing it.

Rather than diet, we install habits of eating the foods we like in ways that will keep us fit. We set up systems to meaningfully and intensely reward the behavior that will make us fit. If you like hamburgers or potatoes or bread or pasta, believe me, there is a way to work it in, and it feels so good when you do, because you not only enjoy the food, but you also enjoy the success. You intensely reward eating those foods only in the fit way, and you install strong habits of eating them only in that way.

In contrast, with dieting, most people deny themselves what they like to eat, and then, after a while, they eat them again in ways that make them fat. And they enjoy it so much! It is such a pleasure and so rewarding! They install incredibly tenacious habits, or programs, to crave and eat what they like only in the ways that make them fat! Dieting, because it is so unpleasant, becomes repulsive. We had literally brainwashed ourselves to be addicted to behaviors that made us fat and repelled by behaviors that made us fit.

In contrast, with The Anderson Method, while we are losing the weight, we learn how to eat absolutely everything we will ever want to eat, in ways that will keep us fit. Rather than trying to avoid foods we like, we build habits of eating them only in fit ways. And by using conditioning techniques, we are not relying solely on will to create this. We are drawing on that inner power that conditioning taps, so that we are *driven* to act in these healthy ways. When we enjoy what we like to eat in ways that keep us fit, not only do we experience the pleasure of the food, but we do it without guilt or shame, and we mentally experience the pleasure of our success. We experience the pleasure of winning, and we enjoy the mental forecasting of our success. We imagine the result of what we are doing, what it's like to live at our target weight, what we are doing at our target weight, what we are wearing at our target weight, how good it feels.

Can you eat everything you like and lose weight? Just about.

A few foods *are* totally incompatible with life and health, like the 800 calorie hamburgers, 2,000 calorie steak dinners, and 1,500 calorie sundaes. So, we need to say goodbye to those forever, because if you have them once, and there is pleasure, you will create the drive and motivation to do it again. (A behavior that is rewarded **will be repeated.**) So, with the behaviors that make us fat, we will never again do them, not even once. No more overeating. We link overeating and the foods and behaviors of overeating with the pain of obesity, the sore knees and feet, the acid reflux, the tight clothes, the stretch marks. We imagine that deep fried onions or potatoes are actually cooked in the grease saved from the bottom of garbage cans. We imagine that the jelly donuts are filled with maggots. We imagine that the 800 calorie hamburgers are filled with artery clogging chemicals (they are) that will start lining our mouths and all our tissues with festering disease the moment we were to bite into one. Some foods are so incompatible with health that we would be better off to never consider them edible.

But, we *can* have hamburgers, steak dinners, and ice cream. There are healthy versions of all of those. We can train ourselves to have them in ways and amounts that are right for us, ways that are "undereating." We can install the habits to enjoy them only in ways to keep us fit. And we can strengthen those habits using that same force from within that drove us to fail in the past.

Conditioning is power. It can help you to call on desire, craving, and repulsion to bring you what you want, rather than what you dread.

Explaining the intricacies of the conditioning methodology and training is not possible in a book like this, nor is the training experience the same as reading about it. But for some, who don't need teachers and coaches, just understanding the mechanics and power of this phenomenon will give them the opportunity to begin training on their own. Perhaps today you can begin linking the pain of obesity to a Big Mac or hot fudge sundae and the joy of your dream-come-true to eating what you like in quantities and frequencies that make you lose weight.

Conditioning power, when used to build healthy habits, or addictions, can be a miraculous ally to the will.

CHAPTER 7

The Power of Thought, The Word, and Imagination

Cognitive Behavior Therapy (CBT) is the most significant innovation in psychotherapy since Sigmund Freud. Maybe it is even more significant than Freud. It is the form of psychotherapy developed from "cognitive" psychology, which focuses on thought, otherwise known as cognition.

While traditional western medicine looks to the body and medicine for answers, and behaviorists look at the observable behavior of "organisms," the cognitive psychologists focus on our thoughts, those intangible mental "things" we can't touch or observe, like the psyche itself.

Western science demands objective verifiable proof of things, so the very "reality" or existence of psyche (mind or soul), or thought, was doubted by many of my early psychology teachers. The brain was real, they said, because we could dissect it and see it— but thought? That was not so easy to determine. Some of my early teachers said that the "mind" and "thought" were just abstract concepts, like side effects; they were transient by-products of the chemical and electrical activity of "matter," which they said was the "real" stuff. Matter was real, but those other things were not. They were like dreams, appearing real, but evaporating and disappearing, while the matter did not.

Now, after an additional forty years of study and experience, I think my early teachers were wrong. While we can't see thoughts and psyche, I think *they* are the underlying reality that brings the other into being. I think those early teachers had it all backwards.

~

Cognitive Behavior Therapy, what may be thought of as a kind of "thought management," has been most significant in treating depression, and it is in this context that we can easily and clearly demonstrate the way that thought generates the reality of our world.

We know that depression exists on several dimensions. We commonly think of depression as being a profoundly sad and discouraged mood that we can't get out of. Maybe we lost a job or a loved one and took it real hard. It's a sad emotion.

But depression is not just a sad mood brought on by bad events.

When a person is severely depressed, they can have physical symptoms, such as insomnia or hypersomnia, body pain, weepiness, slow (retarded) reactions, lack of energy, and appetite disturbance. Physically, depression exists also as a malfunction of the brain, where the normal operation of the brain, via neurotransmitters, is out of whack. It is described as a "chemical imbalance," where the chemical neurotransmitters, such as serotonin, are too low.

When the brain function is restored, by medication that improves the operation of neurotransmission, the symptoms go away! Not only do the physical symptoms improve, but the person's mood gets better, too! Depression is not just a mental disorder. It is a disease of the body, treated by prescribing medication.

Of course, there is the mental component of depression: the sadness, the inability to enjoy anything, the black thoughts. A depressed person may be hopeless and have suicidal thoughts, unable to think that things will ever get better no matter how hard you may try to point out good reasons to expect that they will. They are just stuck, seeing things only one way, the black way. And it is impressive to witness the changes that occur after several weeks on an anti-depressant medication. Recovering patients are sometimes mystified themselves, unable to understand why they thought the way they did before the "chemical imbalance" was corrected in their brain. The dramatic effectiveness of medications would lead one to think that the physical condition creates the mental, the mood and the thoughts. But wait. Don't jump to conclusions.

Research shows that Cognitive Behavior Therapy is just as effective as drugs in treating depression.

How does CBT work?

Usually people think that bad events cause the bad feelings. You get a flat tire on the way to an important meeting in the morning, and it ruins the whole day. You think "Why me?" You say to yourself, "Everything rotten happens to me. I never get a break. There's another day shot to hell." You are in a foul mood for the rest of the day, and you think it was caused by the flat tire. Or it could be the phone call or the letter in the mail. There are thousands of events we could use as examples.

CBT says, "Hold on there. Not so fast." It is not the events that cause the bad feelings, but the way we *think* about them. The person in our example has a flat tire and thinks it's the end of the world and has all kinds of negative self-talk, and then they are ready to jump off the bridge.

But not everyone would think of the flat tire the same way.

A different person might say, "If that's the worst thing that happens in my day, I lead a charmed life." They might say a prayer of thanks that it happened in a place where other people could help, or they might be thankful for AAA, or for living in a time of cell phones. They might say, "Other people are in war zones dodging bullets and bombers or being devastated by natural disasters, while I live in relative calm and comfort. I am so lucky!"

The way these two people will feel will be entirely different, yet the event is the same. If the first person changes the way they think about things, so they have a different script when they talk to themselves, then the way they feel will be different, too.

CBT says that the way we feel is not caused by the events, but by the way we *think* of the events. Change the way you think and you change the way you feel.

This technique works remarkably well, and amazingly, when a person can change the way they process experience, change the way they think, they can change the *physical symptoms* of depression, just like the medicine did. *The change in thinking will change the brain chemistry.* So, we should not jump to the conclusion that the physical reality, whether it is the flat tire or the brain chemistry, is what causes the feelings and the thoughts. Maybe *the thoughts are the cause of things.*

Ages ago, Greek philosophers thought so. One teacher, Plato, taught that the material world that we live in may be a result of the thoughts we have, a kind of "projection," cast onto the screen of the material dimension. To illustrate the idea, he told a story about a man in a cave. Imagine that a man was born in a cave and was chained to a spot where he could not see out or even see the entrance. All he could see was a wall illuminated by the sunlight. It was so dark in his cave that he could not even see himself or his keepers, but only the wall and the shadows that played on it because of the activity that occurred in front of the cave entrance.

An entire world of activity passed in front of the cave entrance, but the man grew up seeing only the shadows, and because that was all he could see, he came to believe that the shadows were the only reality that existed. To him, that was all there was. If he saw a shadow of a man, to him, the shadow *was* the man, and the sounds he heard were coming from the shadow. He had no idea that there was another reality outside the cave, the realm of the real things that cast the shadows that he saw.

We are challenged to contemplate the proposal that the world we live in is something like the cave, where we can see only the shadows of the real forms, the thoughts. The thoughts are the real "things" that form the shapes on the walls of our material world. The thoughts are the things that are of real substance and permanence in another realm, while the material forms they cast come and go. Material things are formed of the stuff of the material world, as a result of thoughts, and then disintegrate in time, much like the dreams that seemed so real.

We know that in the realm of feelings and mood, what we think gives rise to feelings. If our self talk is about how our life sucks because our nail broke, we will feel badly, and it is real. But if we stop ourselves and give thanks for all the blessings we can count, we will feel better, and that is real, too. Real feelings come into being and fade away, depending on what we think. Does what we think cause the rest of our reality? Can we change the course of our life, and our body, by changing what we think?

In a word, yes.

For years now, psychotherapists have been training people to create a new reality for themselves by first thinking it, imagining it.

Do you want to be able to speak to large groups? Start here: Spend a little time each day thinking about it, imagining yourself speaking in front of groups like a pro, relaxed and enjoying it, charming them. Imagine the audience enthralled and loving you. See yourself smiling and having a great time, a master of the material and the crowd.

Want to be a great golfer? Start here: Spend a little time each day thinking about it, imagining yourself playing like Tiger Woods. See yourself in slow motion, hitting the ball perfectly, seeing it go exactly where you want it to go. When you actually play, before the shot, imagine the path the ball will take, "see" it going just where you want it.

Want to live the rest of your life at a healthy weight? Start here: Spend a little time each day thinking about it, imagining yourself fit at the weight you want to be. Picture how you'll look, what you'll do, what you'll wear. Daydream about yourself in the clothes you'd like, being active, feeling good, living life at your target weight. Imagine yourself at all the ages of your life that are coming, lean and fit and happy in all of them. Picture yourself eating healthfully, enjoying the foods you like in healthy amounts, easily able to maintain self-control and moderation.

The idea is that the thinking, the *imagining,* gives our mind the instructions of what to create, the directions of where to take us. It is an affirmation of the concept that our thoughts create the reality of our experience. Want your life to be different? Want your body to be different? Start here: Imagine it. Make a habit of thinking of it, imagining it. Think it, and you'll *be* it.

This proposition leads us a bit farther than conservative cognitive psychotherapy does. Well-accepted clinical orthodoxy stands behind the truth that our feelings' states can be created and managed by managing our thinking. We also know that conditions and operations in your body, like blood pressure, heart rate, immune system function, appetite, craving, and perhaps metabolism, too, can be altered simply by altering your habits of thought. But can we alter the operation of reality beyond our skin simply by imagining it? Can we, for instance, think ourselves rich? Can we think ourselves successful in business or career?

For our purposes here (losing weight and getting healthier and happier), we don't have to accept any more of this proposition than the idea that we can change our self, our body and our life, by thinking it into reality. In the course of The Anderson Method, as provided by my therapists, we have a demonstration that will make an *absolute believer* of you, so that you will never again doubt the incredible power of your own thoughts. We can show you how your thoughts instantly begin working, in the real world, to create what you think about, unconsciously and apart from your will. You will never again be careless about what you let yourself think or say to yourself, because you will realize beyond a shadow of a doubt that you are creating your future when you do.

The 2006 movie *The Secret* has led people to think that it has been a secret that your thoughts create your reality. They framed it as "the law of attraction." Many people think it is a new discovery and that mysterious powers have been conspiring to keep this secret from us. Nothing could be further from the truth.

Our great teachers have been trying to drill this into us from day one. We just wouldn't listen or didn't hear.

Do you remember hearing "In the beginning was the word?" This was a lesson from the Christian bible, which was a restating of lessons from the Jewish bible. This lesson is stated in just about every religion and philosophy that you can find. In the holy books of the religion in which I was raised, it is stated, "In the beginning, there was the Word (translated from the original Greek *logos*, meaning thought,) and the Word was with God, and the Word was God. He was in the beginning with God: all things were made through him, and without him was not anything made that was made."

If we listen and look, we will find this lesson taught over and over again: Our thought is the cause. Our reality is brought into being through the thoughts we have, by the thoughts we have. Thought is the divine creative force that is available to us, if only we honor it. We are made by it. We are made of it. It is the God of our life.

Now, what its exact nature *is* is the stuff of religions, science, and philosophies. I would encourage you to look into that subject later, but one thing at a time. We are chiefly concerned here with changing our body and our habits, and the reason for this discussion is to drill into you the immense power of your thought— more powerful than your puny will, more powerful than conditioning and addiction, when it is used in the right way.

The Secret is not a secret, which thankfully, the movie explains, sighting the teachers throughout the ages who have been telling us over and over again to "pay attention."

Today's teachers of cognitive therapy are saying, "Pay attention to your thoughts and words." Stop saying things like "I can never stick to anything. No matter what I do, I can't lose weight." If you do, that's the reality you'll create.

Instead say "I haven't been successful in the past, but if I learn what I need to know, and work to improve my skills, *I will be successful*, just like other people who have had the same problem."

Say "When I develop the habits to eat what I like, in fewer calories than I use, *I will lose weight*, just like every other living thing on the planet." (We'll go over the irrefutable science later in the book. There is a *guaranteed* way to eat where you will lose weight— no ifs, ands, or buts.) Instead, say "I hadn't learned how to control myself to stick to things in the past, but that doesn't mean I can't work at it and learn how it's done. *I can learn how self-control is mastered.*"

Pay attention to your words, and don't utter anything that you don't want to make real in your life.

WE THINK IN WORDS AND IMAGES

Psychology teaches that we think in words and images, mental pictures. Those are the primary forms of our thoughts.

If the holy books have any truth to them, not to mention all the other teachers and therapists, the things we say to ourselves and what we imagine form the reality of our lives and our world.

YOU POWER YOUR WILL WITH THOUGHT

When you imagine, when you picture yourself and your life, you are giving your mind its instructions, and if those images are contrary to your will, your will has no power. The imagination has the power.

If you believe you are destined to fail, then that's what you'll imagine, and something within you will begin working to make it happen. If you believe that you will be fat, no matter what, like others in your family, *that's* what you'll imagine. Then, that's what the creative force in you, the wellspring of the drive we talked about, will make happen. It's a crazy thought, of course. No matter what your genetics, if you eat less calories than you burn, you'll lose weight. It's impossible to stay fat if you eat less than you use. But if you imagine staying fat, it will be next to impossible to behave in a way to make you fit.

With The Anderson Method, you are trained to change the way you think, the words you say to yourself, the way you picture yourself, what you imagine for your future. It is the stuff of hypnosis, cybernetics, and miracles. It is what makes dreams come true.

You are also challenged to make wholesale changes in *all* the words and pictures you pass through your mind— in your beliefs, your philosophy, your way of life.

Do you think that eating out all the time in fancy restaurants is the good life? That eating whatever you feel like is a wonderful joy and luxury? That fast food is convenient and economical? That life should be easy? No, no, no, and no.

Eating out all the time in fancy restaurants is gluttonous and decadent, leading to decay of the body and soul.

Eating whatever you feel like at any time is what makes stretch marks, tight clothes, diabetes, and lost dreams. Like the junkie loving the fix, in the end it brings body rot and destruction, tears and hopelessness. Saying it is the good life is a shameless lie.

Fast food is no more convenient than microwaved low-calorie frozen meals, and far less healthy.

Life is the way it is, and it's what you make of it. There is no one dictating what it should be for you, as if there was some rule somewhere about that. You are allowed to make of it what you can.

What kind of ideas and images do you pass through your mind every day? What TV shows? What books and magazines? What social discussion? What are your friends like?

If you watch shows about the idle and foolish, what lifestyle are you imagining and then creating? If you read trashy books and tabloids, what are you thinking and picturing? If you hang out with drinkers and overeaters, what are you thinking and imagining? What "visions" are you setting your mind on to make of yourself? What have you come to believe is normal? What have you made normal?

If you watch TV, with seventy percent of the ads for food, what are you visualizing, thinking about, and imagining? If you watch cooking shows and talk about recipes all the time, what are you thinking about, imagining, and "attracting?"

You have a set of beliefs about what's OK and what's not OK, and chances are, when you live in the land of the obese, in the culture of the "consumers," it's pretty unhealthy. Do you think getting big portions is a good value at a restaurant? It's not. Getting healthy portions of good food where you know how many calories there are is a good value. Do you think retiring and living a life of leisure is the good life? It's not. Doing what it takes to make a good life for your whole world, as well as yourself, is the good life.

When you truly want to stop being overweight and sick, and you want to have a happier life, it will require changes. But before you can experience changes in your body and behavior, you will need to make changes in the way you think, in what you believe, in how you think of yourself, in what you say to yourself, and in the culture and philosophy you adopt.

Start now by deciding that you'll question and change the way you've been thinking and believing.

When you are told "You deserve a break today," think "I deserve to feel better and eat healthier today."

When you are told that a buffet restaurant is good because you get to eat an unlimited amount, tell them that it reminds you of pigs at a trough. A restaurant is good if it has great food and great service and makes it easy to eat healthfully.

When someone calls you a consumer, say "don't label me a consumer. I'm a producer. I don't diminish the world. I'm a contributor. I make it better."

When someone says it's impossible to live in a fit way, that to function socially, you simply have to have big, festive meals, and eat too much, say "No, that's not true. We can have modest meals and still have a wonderful time."

When someone says it's necessary to drink and have big business lunches to succeed in business, say "No, that's not true. We can eat small. We can meet at other times."

When someone says that your family is fat because of genetics, say "No, that's not true. They were fat because they all ate too much as a lifestyle, by habit. I'm going to break the mold. I was made to be fit and healthy, like all the other species in creation. I am becoming fit, as I was made to be."

Those words and imaginings have power.

As I said, will power is not all it's cracked up to be. There are higher powers at work. When you use your will to engage those powers, then you have a chance.

CHAPTER 8

What's to Eat?

My clients drive people crazy at parties. We seem to eat all the wrong things. We'll have drinks and steak and pizza and desserts. We don't eat just salad and fish and chicken. We don't abstain from the things we like. It doesn't look like we're dieting; but, we *are* losing weight.

"Now, don't cheat!" they'll say. "You've done so good!"

What we do defies their reality. We just love partaking in what we like, what they think is the forbidden fruit. We tell them "This *is* my diet!" while they look in bewilderment at our plates of the "wrong" things.

Different ideas come to mind when you talk about dieting. Most people think of it as a different way of eating that you do for a while to lose weight. You "diet" to lose weight, and then when you're done, you go back to normal.

This does no good. In fact, it makes us worse, helping us develop more overeating habits. It makes us crave and overvalue some foods, and it conditions us to overeat without control, through an inadvertent application of those behavioral principles I spoke of earlier. While you diet, you engage in a punitive exercise of deprivation and eating in a way you don't like. It's a form of aversion "therapy." It trains you to hate and be repelled by eating in ways to make you lose weight. Then you stop dieting, and you start thoroughly enjoying eating what you like, without limit, which conditions you to overeat and triggers drives to addict you to compulsive overeating. Dieting, in this sense, doesn't work— or I should say that it makes things worse. It's a perfect system to create an overeater, a food addict.

With The Anderson Method, we have no diets of what you have to eat, and what you can't eat. If you are going to succeed, you have to like what you eat, and you have to learn how to eat what you like. With my method, you don't eat things you don't like, and you eat all the things you *do* like, in ways where you won't become overweight. Believe me, there are very few things that must be given up for all time.

Sometimes when people use the word "dieting," they mean eating responsibly or eating with self-control. When they "diet," they eat in a healthy, self-controlled way, and when they are not "dieting," they practice no self-control. They eat with wild abandon, sometimes off on a rampage, compulsively, continuously, "foraging," and bingeing.

With my method, there are no lists of foods that are OK or not OK and no rules about when to eat. There are no silly edicts about chewing twenty-eight times, or against eating and watching TV at the same time. There's nothing about avoiding all food that's white, or about needing to eat a big breakfast. You can eat after 7:00 p.m., if that's what you want.

But you do learn self-control. You *can*, and to succeed, we need to practice this self-control for the rest of our lives. This *can* be done, when it is rewarding, rather than punitive and repulsive. It can become habitual, and enjoyable, and self-sustaining. Our goal is not as much about learning how to lose weight or diet, as it is about learning how to eat and learning how to control your weight. It's about changing what you do when you act natural, what you feel like doing. It's about making eating with self-control what you feel like doing.

We will not solve our problem by doing something weird for a while and then going back to "normal." The old "normal" is what made us fat. And "dieting" is what made our "normal" behavior worse.

To succeed, we need to learn how to eat, to *undereat*, not "diet." We need to learn how to live in a way where we will lose the weight and then control it. To succeed, we need to do this forever. To succeed, there is no going back to "normal."

You will succeed by getting trained, or by training yourself, to eat what you like, and everything you like, in a way that will make you lose your excess weight and keep you at the weight you want to be. There *is* a way. It *can* be done. My clients do it every day. You can do it, too.

To lay the groundwork for this, you will need to become acquainted, or reacquainted, with the facts related to weight control from the physical sciences. So, prepare for a little bit of scholarly study.

WHAT WE KNOW FOR SURE ABOUT HOW TO LOSE WEIGHT

There is no mystery about the physics of weight control.

Your body is a machine that runs on fuel— the food we eat. If you live in a way where you take in more fuel in any given month than you burn, you'll store it, in the form of fat, and gain weight. If you burn more than you've taken in, you'll burn some of your stored fat and lose weight. If you live in a way where at the end of the month you've only taken in the amount you burn, you'll stay the same. This is irrefutable, reliable, science.

The fuel in food is measured in calories. A calorie is the amount of energy required to heat a gram of water one degree Celsius.

Calories are units of energy measurement, like the BTUs you see on gas grills. The label on the grill tells you how much energy the grill can consume and put out, for instance, forty thousand BTUs. The BTU (British Thermal Unit) is the amount of energy it takes to heat a gallon of water one degree Fahrenheit. We measure energy for gas grills in BTUs, and we measure energy for people in calories.

If you eat more calories than you need, you'll gain weight. Period. The only way to lose weight is to eat fewer calories than you need. Period. There is no avoiding this reality. It is no more avoidable than the law of gravity. If you try to fight it or fool it, you will lose. You can only succeed by living with it rather than trying to get around it.

How many calories does your body need? Your body didn't come with a label like the gas grill, but it is a simple thing to find out how much energy you burn in the course of a day. They call it your "metabolic rate." It's almost like the mileage rating on a car. If you're a six foot tall man of average activity, your metabolic rate is about 2,700 calories per day. If you are a five foot, four inch woman of average activity, your metabolic rate is about 1,800 calories per day. (Sporty, little, efficient cars use less than big, lumbering SUVs.)

We have very accurate methods to estimate a person's metabolic rate. Incredibly, most of the information you will get on the internet about your metabolic rate is horribly inaccurate, even from sources you'd assume were legitimate. Also a surprise: Many doctors and even "nutritionists" are completely mistaken about how to estimate a person's metabolic rate. If you wanted to get an actual clinical measurement, that can be obtained, too. There are several methods, using devices called "calorimeters," which can physically and scientifically measure how much fuel you burn. Your doctor can refer you to an endocrinologist who can arrange a test, if you'd like an exact measure of your individual rate. (If you think you have a strange metabolism,

I strongly advise you to get tested. Most of the time, you'll find out that you don't have an unusually slow metabolism, but some do, and they need medical treatment. Those who are normal, but who were convinced that their body had a "slow metabolism," need a reality check so they can be confident that eating fewer calories will have the desired effect.)

There is no way to alter your metabolic rate if you don't have a metabolic disorder. There are no pills or foods that will speed up your metabolism. Exercise will burn more calories, but not really that much, relative to what you can eat. Exercise is useless as a help to lose weight if you don't control your eating; and people who control their eating to lose weight can do just fine without exercise. Exercise is a separate health issue, and it is really unrelated to the obesity problem we have. Our weight problems are because of the way we eat, and the solution is in changing the way we eat.

We can measure the fuel value in all the foods we eat, and there are countless sources of data available, so we can know very accurately the number of calories in all the foods we eat and the number of calories we put in our body each day and over time.

Clients engaging in The Anderson Method go through a training process where they end up eating what they like, habitually, in the amounts of calories to maintain the weight they want to be. It's a lot of work at first, but the goal is to make it so you have a new "normal," not by eating diet stuff, but by eating what you like in a way to get the weight off and keep it off.

Clients learn to *undereat*, rather than overeat. They develop a way to eat during the week and on the weekend, a way to eat at restaurants, a way to go to parties, a way to have Thanksgiving (including the pumpkin pie). The goal is for undereating to become the new normal, so that when you do what feels good, you are doing what gets you to your target weight and keeps you there. Rather than doing without things, like ice cream or bacon, for instance, we develop a way to work it into a healthy behavioral pattern that will keep us fit. We train in it until it becomes our new normal, and any other way would be uncomfortable.

It's not rocket science. It's simple in concept, though complex in execution, and it is irrefutable and utterly reliable. You will lose weight, without question.

There are many details of the therapy that are complex and beyond the scope of this book, but you will be exposed to the essence that is at the core.

NOTHING NEW UNDER THE SUN

You may be wondering "What about carbs and fat, and what you eat at night turning to fat?" Let me help you change a bad habit you probably have, hopefully forever.

The physics and nutrition science we are involving here is not subject to opinion, like opinions about what are the best foods to eat. It has not really changed in the last twenty years.

These facts regarding your weight being a result of the number of calories you eat are not up for debate. There are scientists who study these things at all our universities, and they all agree. It doesn't really matter what time of day you take in your calories, or even what day. It doesn't really matter if you get your calories from carbs or protein, or junk food or diet food. If you eat more calories, on average, than you use, you will gain weight. Period. Accumulate 3500 calories of excess, and you've gained a pound of fat.

If you eat fewer calories than you use, by undereating, you'll lose weight. Period.

Stop reading goofy articles by people who are not qualified. Stop listening to diet gossip. Rid your brain of all the nonsense you've accumulated.

If you want a factual answer about the science involved here, go to an R.D., a Registered Dietician. They are the scientists who have specialized in the physical sciences regarding food, your body, and weight. They will tell you "a calorie is a calorie is a calorie."

I trust R.D.s regarding the science, though I still don't like them telling me what to eat and when, which they seem to like to do. I know there are reasons they think their way of eating is better, but it often has nothing to do with what I want, which is my happy successful weight control. They are experts in the physical sciences, not psychology and behavioral science. So, you don't have to believe all their opinions about how to live, but trust them with the physics. If you live in a way where your calorie balance is *negative*, because your habits automatically make it so in the long run, you'll master your weight control. You will never be overweight again. That's what my clients are able to do with the practice of my method. It just becomes the way they live their life, week in, week out.

CHAPTER 9

Mysteries Answered

How many times have you wondered what's wrong when you observe your skinny friends eating the same or worse than you?

When I was fat, it drove me crazy. It just didn't seem fair. It didn't seem that I ate any worse than anyone else, but I got fat. They could eat all the things I couldn't, and they had no problem. How could this be, if my metabolism was not screwed up? (And the doctors claimed it wasn't.)

When you look at two people, and one is a perfect 120 pounds at five feet, four inches, and the other is two-hundred and fifty pounds at the same height, everyone assumes that the overweight person eats twice as much, right?

Let me straighten out some misconceptions.

Your metabolic rate depends, more than any other factor, on your height or muscle mass, not your weight. When you get overweight, you have more fat, not muscle, so your metabolic rate is not much different than when you were not overweight. Two women, each five feet, four inches, will have very similar metabolic rates, about 1,800 calories per day, even though one is 120 and the other is 250.

If the skinny one eats an 1,800 calorie average, she'll stay right where she is. What happens if the fat one eats like the skinny one?

Most people will think that if the fat one eats like the skinny one, she'll get skinny, too. Wrong. She'll stay right where she is, just like the skinny one will stay where *she* is.

The conception that fat people must eat so much more to maintain that weight is an absolute fallacy. In fact, if the skinny one is lots more active because the fat one is limited and sedentary, the skinny one may burn more! In that case, the fat one might eat *less* than the skinny one to maintain her weight. Chances are she *is* less active and *does* eat less than her skinny friend and is still overweight! All the while her skinny friend eats more than she does and stays 120 pounds! How unfair!

So it's true that my skinny friends got to eat whatever they wanted, and they had no problem, as long as they ate whatever they wanted in caloric quantities within their "budget."

I, on the other hand, tried to eat less of the "bad" foods, felt deprived, then felt guilty and like a failure when I did eat them. I gained weight, not because of the "bad" foods, but because my total consumption with all the calories counted (including the diet food) was "over budget."

SO, HOW'D I GET OVERWEIGHT IF I ATE LIKE THEM?

Most of us get overweight over a period of time. We eat an average of a bit more calories than we burn. It's cumulative.

For instance, imagine that, by some miracle, you were one of the people who made it to early adulthood without a weight problem. By dumb luck, you just happened to form habits where your caloric consumption matched your burn. You're five feet, four inches, 120 pounds. But then, your friend convinces you to drink a big glass of fortified orange juice every morning, a health drink. It has calcium and vitamin C, and it's orange juice, for goodness sake! It's good for you!

So, you start drinking this big glass of orange juice in addition to what you normally ate that kept you skinny. You start accumulating two hundred calories a day surplus on your body, which isn't that much, if you look only at that one day. It's a new blob of body fat only about the size of two tablespoons. But then you add to it the next day, and the next, and so on.

By the time a month has gone by, you've gained almost two pounds. It's not really that noticeable, and in *your* mind, you are not overeating. You're not eating any differently than you always have.

By the time a year goes by, you've gained twenty pounds. So you go to the doctor to find out what's wrong with your metabolism. He says there's nothing wrong, that you eat too much, which is an insult, so you find a new doctor. You don't change how you eat because you don't think you eat incorrectly, and five years later, you're one hundred pounds overweight! *On a glass of orange juice!*

Or worse, you go on a diet, and when you're done, you can't wait to have all those things you've done without, and they're so good! And something in you now drives you to eat goodies without restriction, which you never did before, and you hate even the thought of dieting. With that, you'd be two hundred pounds overweight in a couple of years, instead of one hundred. But you can't stand it, so every once in a while you try to diet, and sometimes you do lose some weight. But then, when you stop the diet, you always gain back more than you lost.

BUT IF I JUST EAT RIGHT AGAIN, I'LL BE OK, RIGHT?

No, and here's why.

Suppose after gaining one hundred pounds, you finally figure out that the problem is the orange juice (or a few drinks, or a little ice cream every night).

You think "I'll just go back to eating the way I did when I was 120 all those years, and I'll be fine."

Wrong. When you go back to eating what maintained 120, all you'll do is maintain 220! Remember, your metabolic rate depends on your height, not your weight. If anything, you probably burn less, because you're not as active.

So, once you've packed it on, eating "right" won't fix things. It will just keep you where you now are.

OTHER INSIDIOUS WAYS WE GAIN WEIGHT

HAVE A BABY

The doctor says "You need to put on some weight. I want you to gain twenty-five pounds. Eat cake and ice cream."

So, now you have license to eat, and you gain fifty pounds. You have the baby. Then you're still forty pounds overweight, and you have conditioned yourself into a cake and ice cream addiction. You'll be lucky to avoid being four hundred as a result of his advice.

But, you strive to get back to the good eating you had before the baby, and you think that then the weight should go.

Nope. If you're now 160, and you go back to the good eating that had you maintain 120, you'll just stay 160....until the next baby. Then you'll be 200. God forgive you if you have three!

BE AN ATHLETE

This is a rotten trick that gets played on lots of men, as well as women.

Imagine that a guy is into sports, and all year long he plays on the school's teams. Football, baseball, basketball, soccer, all through high school and college. Every day, he is out on the field, burning up an extra 1,500 calories a day in intense exercise. And over the years, he develops the eating habits to support those needs.

Now, when he graduates, he starts working in a bank, but his eating habits have hardened like a plaster cast. Even though he cuts back, he gains an enormous amount of weight, fifty to one hundred pounds in a year! Everyone figures he must have a metabolic disease. Nope. He graduated.

GET MARRIED

Imagine that you are a woman, five foot, four inches at 120, with a burn rate of 1,800. Miraculously, you've managed to keep your girlish figure into your thirties. Then, you marry a guy six feet tall with a burn rate of 2,700 calories.

So, now you're living together. He has a drink; you have a drink. He has a dessert; you have a dessert. If you add only two drinks and two desserts a week to what you had been doing, that will be twenty extra pounds in one year, one hundred pounds overweight in five years. The bum!

GROW UP

Imagine you survive your youth and make it to middle age, and miraculously, you are one of those people who never had a weight problem. But now you are older, and your body starts changing. Your metabolism slows down. Not much, but say it shrinks by five percent. Now, instead of breaking even, you start accumulating one hundred calories of fat a day. It's not much, but it's cumulative. After a year, you've gained ten pounds. After five years, it's fifty pounds. After eight years, it's eighty pounds! And it's so unfair! You don't overeat! You're not like those fat people whom you assumed were so flawed. Guess what? You are now one of us. You have eating habits that make you fat, and they are hard to change. And when you try to diet, you fail, and you can't control yourself, and it gets worse. Your desire and urges get the best of you. You are a food addict.

LIVE IN AMERICA

Remember, our energy balance doesn't have to be too far out of whack to cause a big problem. A glass of orange juice at two hundred calories can cause a gain of one hundred pounds over a five-year period.

Eat 3,500 calories over what you need and you'll gain a pound. And you won't get rid of it, even if you eat "right," even if you eat just what the dietician says. It will sit there and wait for another to join it the next time you eat more than you need.

You could eat perfect all week long, eating just what the dietician tells you, and you "cheat" only once a week with a hot fudge sundae and gain twenty-five pounds a year. Think about it. *You could follow the dietician's diet all week long, cheat only once a week with a 1,500 calorie sundae, and become one hundred pounds overweight in four years.*

Eat five hundred calories more than you need a day, and you'll be fifty pounds overweight in a year, 250 pounds overweight in five years.

Look around. McDonald's newly introduced hamburger is eight hundred calories. Many pastries, donuts, and bagels are about five hundred calories. Denny's Grand Slam breakfast is 1,100 calories. Some of the fancy "coffee" shop drinks are over five hundred calories, up to seven hundred. A bowl of ice cream can be five hundred calories. A drink with an umbrella can be about five hundred calories. Many of the steaks they serve in steakhouses are over one thousand calories. The bloomin' onion "appetizer" is about two thousand calories!

How difficult do you think it would be to slip in five hundred calories a day over what you burn? It would be easy, wouldn't it? That's how easy it could be to become one hundred or even two hundred pounds overweight.

Look around. Look at the way food is advertised and glorified in the media, and how food is sold as the satisfier of every human need. Food is a part of every shopping experience, every night out, every fair and festival, every holiday, even church and religious experiences. Look how food is sold as a form of recreation, as entertainment, as the answer to social success, even as the answer to weight control! Ha! Want to lose weight? The food companies have the answer! Eat something! (In 1978, H.J. Heinz, the ketchup company, bought Weight Watchers and today makes all the Weight Watcher Smart Ones foods.)

The food merchants are stalking you. They are stalking your children. They are selling food as recreation, as entertainment, as fashion, as a personal statement, as the answer to all manner of emotional needs, in the schools, as well as in your living room through the TV.

The tobacco companies got caught a while back mercilessly manipulating the nicotine in cigarettes and lying about it. They got caught marketing to kids and lying about it. They got caught knowing that they were selling us a cancer-causing product and lying about it. They had an addictive drug product and a market of addicts. It was a pusher's dream. But they got caught and sued and made to pay for their sins, and then they complained it would put them out of business. So what did they do?

They went into the food business, I kid you not.

In 1985, R.J. Reynolds (Camel, Winstons, Salems, and others) acquired Nabisco Brands (Oreos, Chips Ahoy, Fig Newtons, Ritz Crackers, and many other food products you are familiar with).

In 1988, Philip Morris (Marlboro, Virginia Slims, and others— the largest tobacco company in the world) acquired Kraft Foods (Kraft Cheese, Maxwell House coffee, Kool-Aid, Oscar Mayer, and many other products you are familiar with).

Since then, the trading of ownership of these companies is hard to follow, but remember that industry is populated by people, and in this case, the guys who spent millions and millions of dollars on sophisticated advertising (brainwashing) to get us addicted to consuming a product that was killing us.

The guys who made their money getting us hooked on cigarettes are now doing it with food.

Consider how easy it is to overeat five hundred calories a day (one donut, or one bagel, or one small fries, or a half a burger, or a Starbuck's "coffee.") This little bit extra would result in a gain of fifty pounds a year! When you consider that, it's a miracle we all aren't six hundred pounds! If we keep going the way we've been going, it's only a matter of time. Today, two-thirds of us are overweight. The government's CDC says we have an obesity *epidemic*. Where will we be in another ten to twenty years? Will we all be obese?

We are addicted to our way of life, to our consumerism, to overeating, and to our food. Changing will require a great effort. But we *can* change. You *can* become an undereater, a contributor rather than a consumer.

Don't worry about everyone else changing. Change yourself. Change yourself, and you'll change your world.

When you change how you eat and how you think, it will transform your life and your body. When you change yourself, it will have an impact on everyone around you, on every *thing* around you. You can have a world-changing impact just by changing yourself.

You may have initially wanted to lose weight only for your own personal reasons, but if you are successful, you will give a great gift to the world. Your well-being will be contagious. You can begin your own trend away from consuming, which ruins us individually, as well as the planet, and you can lead the charge to save us, simply by focusing on solving your own weight problem. Start taking care of yourself, your thinking, your habits, and your body, and the effect will spread.

CHAPTER 10

Undereating

In behaviorism, one of the key principles in learning and habituation is *modeling*. Human beings have an innate capacity and tendency to copy a model. This is the natural way we learn or acquire many of our traits and behaviors, and we can take advantage of this phenomenon to succeed in weight control. We can intentionally seek out models who display the real world results we'd like, like being thin. Then, we can intentionally engage in techniques to adopt the characteristics of the model that cause those results.

There are some almost magical kinds of techniques that we'll talk about later, but the simplest example is simply copying.

You look for people who are fit, and you find out what they're doing. You study them. Then you copy how they act, what they do.

The body is a result of the behavior we have. There's no mystery there. If you behave the way they do, you'll get the same result in your body as they do. You find out how they live and think and see if it's something you can adopt yourself.

There are lots of facets and exquisite details of behavior you can catalogue, but you can sum up the totality in one word: They *undereat,* rather than overeat. They eat less than they need, rather than more than they need. Rather than intend to eat all they can and try to see how much they can get away with, they *intend* to eat less than they need.

That's where to start, with that simple intention.

In this chapter, I'll describe some of the target behaviors that we've identified as behaviors that make a person an undereater. We identify and define the habits, the behaviors, the ways that they act and think, that make them fit. If we can get ourselves to act in the ways that make people fit, we'll get the same result as they get: a fit body.

I will not try to explain here how we get ourselves to build these habits, all the details of the training experience, or "brainwashing," as some clients call it. The knowledge of the behavioral traits alone will be of immense value.

CONSCIOUS EATING

Many years ago, when I was a very overweight young professional, I was attending a business luncheon, and I learned a great lesson from an older woman sitting across the table from me.

I had been overweight and struggling with the problem for years, and at this particular time, I was not dieting. I was doing what I did when I wasn't dieting, which was overeating and feeling bad about it.

At the Exchange Club weekly luncheon, I was having my usual: a little steak, a little side of spaghetti, a salad, and coffee. A few minutes earlier, I had had a bloody Mary, as it was the custom to "schmooze" a bit before the luncheon. Then, while the speaker spoke, we'd have dessert, usually a little piece of cake or dish of ice cream.

Little did I know that the "lunch" I had was about 1,500 calories.

In my career as a chronically overweight dieter, I had never counted a calorie except for diet food. I had no idea what calories were in real food.

After years of being overweight and dieting, I had come to hate the word "calorie," and I hated dieting. I wanted a way to lose weight without counting calories; I hated it so much. I wanted a way where I didn't have to do any hateful work. I thought if someone else could just give me the meals already counted, I'd win. Of course, even if I lost weight on the diet, I gained it all back and more when I stopped dieting.

So, here I was, eating my little steak (OK by Atkins), and I spotted this older skinny lady across the table eating a salad, and she said something to the lady next to her about the number of calories in what they were serving and "saving" her calories for later.

I was incensed! *How dare* she be talking about calories when she was skinny, with obviously no reason to count calories!

So, I said something like "Why are you concerned about calories? You don't have a weight problem."

She said "Young man, why do you think I don't have a weight problem?" Then she proceeded to tell me that she doesn't have a weight problem anymore because she doesn't eat anything without knowing the calories in it, and she doesn't eat more calories than she needs to maintain her weight. It turned out that at one time, she had been eighty pounds more in her "past life."

I don't think I said much more after that. But I thought about it.

One of the things that all successful people do is "conscious eating." They don't put anything in their mouths without knowing how many calories it is. They never, ever, eat unconsciously, closing their eyes to what they are putting in their mouths and swallowing.

For a long time, I resisted this, thinking that it was a hideous, awful way to live. I had counted calories a little, and it was so painful I couldn't stand it.

I have since learned that it is a lot of work at first, but done right, it's not that bad, and it can become easy. That's one of the things our training helps with.

We start out just counting, and making an effort *not* to eat any differently for at least a week— to just eat the way we usually do and become aware of the calories in what we usually eat. What an eye-opener! What an education!

That's the beginning, and we don't try to make any changes in the actual eating and eating habits until we employ some of the other tools we learn about.

Undereaters, whether they are trained in my method or they are self-trained, never eat unconsciously. They know what they are eating. They never eat anything without thinking about it. They know the calories. They know the calories they've eaten that day.

This is one of the behaviors they have that we copy, and we have a way of learning to do it that is not so hideous. In fact, believe it or not, it can become enjoyable, even fun.

PLANNING AHEAD

People who have succeeded in losing weight and keeping it off don't eat spontaneously. They have a plan. They know ahead of time what they are going to do for the day, and what they are going to eat.

This is another idea that I found hideous when I was fat. I wanted to be a free spirit. "Don't fence me in!" I thought. I didn't like structure imposed, and I resisted the whole idea of the work and oppression of developing plans that made me lose weight. It seemed overwhelming and cold and stark, compared with my preferred lifestyle of ease and comfort. I thought I could only succeed if someone else did the work and planning for me. Wrong.

With The Anderson Method, we have a way of easing you into the work so it is not quite so awful, and after a while, it's all habit, so it isn't really much work at all.

It won't always be so much work, but to succeed, there will always be planning.

I know every day before I leave the house in the morning, what I'll be eating for the day. I look forward to it. I am still a food addict of sorts, and I thoroughly enjoy everything I eat, and I enjoy looking forward to it, too. But I no longer overeat.

Planning ahead is certainly important to get the calories right, but the most important benefit is that it engages those powers of imagining and expectation we referred to earlier. Later on, I'll explain more about Therapeutic Psychogenics, but for now, suffice it to say that planning ahead sets your subconscious on the task of leading you to eat in the way that makes you successful, so that something inside you leads you and drives you there, instead of taking you in some other direction.

Undereaters know what kind of eating takes them where they want to be. They enjoy it, they look forward to it, and they plan on it.

NO DIETS

People who have successfully maintained a healthy weight after having had a weight problem don't diet, and didn't really diet in the traditional sense to lose the weight. They made permanent lifestyle changes.

If we are going to solve this problem, the main thing we need to learn is how to live in a way so that we don't gain weight. We need habits that we'll practice forever, that will keep us fit. So, doing something for a while, even if we lose weight, will do no good if our lifestyle and habitual way of living makes us gain weight.

So, we need to keep eating what we know we'll want to eat for the rest of our lives, *while* we are losing weight, instead of doing without. There *is* a way. We need to keep the activities we know we'll want to engage in for the rest of our lives. We need to learn to work our foods and activities into a lifestyle that will keep us fit. There is a way this can be done, so that over time, you'll have developed a new way of eating, a new way of doing things that includes what you like, that you can live with.

MEALS AND FASTING

The first time I honestly started counting my calories, and I ate as I usually did, I was shocked. I found that on many days, I took in most of my calories when I wasn't eating!

That is to say, my "snacking" counted for more calories than my meals.

I'd sit down and have a coffee with someone and have a donut or a cookie (five hundred calories). I'd get a bag of Doritos to munch on as I drove around (1,500 calories). I'd have a bit of ice cream while I watched TV (one thousand calories in six trips to the fridge during a movie). I'd have a candy bar or bag of cashews in the checkout line while shopping (250 to five hundred calories).

That first week, I realized that if my life was an unstructured flow of spontaneous eating, there would be no hope whatsoever of controlling my weight, not to mention losing weight. The typical doctor's diet was one thousand or 1200 calories a day! Some of my snacks were more than that all by themselves! When I "grazed," or "snacked," it was so easy to accumulate a surplus of calories over my metabolic rate that there was no hope at all, unless I stopped eating whenever I felt like it.

Years before, one of my thin friends once remarked "You're eating all the time." I wasn't eating *all* the time, of course, but *he* ate only at meals, and he thought my way of living was bizarre. Of course, I thought *he* was kind of strange. I thought it was normal to just eat something whenever you felt like it, or whenever it appeared.

In America, it *is* normal to eat all the time, and that's one of our problems. It's normal, but it's killing us, and we need to change. It is simply not OK to eat the entire time we are awake, like one continuous meal.

Undereaters have a couple of times a day that they take in food. Those are their meals. The rest of the time, they don't eat.

My thin friend would say things like "I already had breakfast" if we were offered donuts, while I thought to myself, "What's that got to do with anything?"

In the afternoon, he would pass up chips and dip saying "I'm having dinner pretty soon," while I thought to myself, "So what?"

To me, eating was a pastime, a recreational activity that you engaged in spontaneously. But to him, there were definite rules, and you simply did not eat unless you were having a meal.

He would say to me "You just ate a little while ago. How can you be hungry?"

It was a question I didn't understand. Eating always seemed like a good idea. I always had an appetite. How could anyone *not* want to eat something that was good?

He would intentionally abstain from food and wait until he was having a meal, as if he was "fasting" until his next meal.

Undereaters have several discreet bits of time during the day they sit down and eat. Those are called "meals." The rest of the time they are fasting; they eat nothing.

So, we copy them. It turns out that it doesn't matter when you have your meals or what's in them. My clients have all sorts of different styles. Some have two meals a day, some four, some six. It doesn't matter. Some have breakfast, some don't. Some eat late at night. It doesn't matter. But they only eat at the meals they've planned on, and the rest of the time, they *fast*, and they take in nothing but non-caloric drinks.

Making it black and white or on/off like this has advantages. The eating switch is "on" a few times a day, and you pay attention to the calories. The rest of the time, the switch is off, and there's nothing to count.

Thinking of it as *fasting* has an advantage, too. Rather than "doing without," or doing nothing, you are actively engaged in a substantial activity. You are thoroughly occupied, like a religious zealot, doing something of great importance, which, of course, you are. You are burning calories, losing weight, and achieving your heart's desire. You are fasting, and becoming the size and weight you want to be.

WORKING, RESTING— TENSING, RELAXING

Generations ago, we feasted on occasion. We'd work hard, be frugal, and every once in a while, we'd feast. Thanksgiving. Holy days.

Today, we feast every day. And it's killing us.

Lean people don't feast all the time. They do it occasionally. The rest of the time, they are pretty austere in their eating. It's a good practice to copy.

We will not have to give up good food, or enjoying it, or even looking forward to it. But we are going to stop having feasts every day with all the trimmings.

We take advantage of a dynamic in our psyche where we find enjoyment and tolerance through the play between extremes. We are able to tolerate a job that is perhaps not much fun because we get weekends off. TGIF!

We find delight in days off precisely because we don't have them every day. Have you ever talked with a retired person who has gone back to work because the "days off" lost their magic? They'll say things like "The weekends weren't special anymore."

Great pleasure can be experienced in the play between tension and relaxing. You might not think sitting down is an exquisite pleasure, but if you've ever been on your feet a few hours beyond the point where you can stand it, you'll find that sitting down can be the most enjoyable of experiences. Likewise, you can tolerate an ugly job, like walking many blocks back to where the car was parked, as long as you can stop and rest at times.

So, as undereaters in The Anderson Method, we undereat severely during the week, Monday through Friday, nose to the grindstone, and then, TGIF, we relax a bit on the weekend. And we do this not just to lose weight, but to maintain a healthy weight. And we do it as a lifetime habit.

When you become aware of the calories in some of the foods you like, in restaurant meals, in drinks and foods you'd have at parties, and you compare those numbers with what you need to do to lose weight, you'll see that it is impossible to have many of them. If you go to a birthday party, how do you get a glass of wine (one hundred calories), a decent steak (550 calories), and a piece of cake (350 calories) into a one thousand calorie day? That's one thousand right there, and we haven't accounted for what else you'd have in that meal or any other food for the day. Impossible!

But remember that the body doesn't operate on a twenty-four hour a day clock, and even a tiny woman with a metabolic rate of 1,500 calories has a weekly "budget" of 10,500 calories. That means that if she ate one thousand calories per day for five days, she'd have to eat over five thousand calories on the weekend to gain weight!

We can figure out how to eat pretty much anything we want, but we can only avoid getting obese if we keep it real low five days a week.

Undereaters, as a lifestyle, for the rest of their lives, eat very austerely all week long. On the weekend, they get to eat just about anything they want. Then they go back to work every Monday. They don't feast and party day after day.

And guess what? The food tastes better than it ever has. You'll enjoy it more than you ever have. If you can eat everything you like all the time, it loses its magic, just like the weekends that weren't special anymore for the retirees.

So, one of the most important undereating behaviors to copy is the practice of eating like a health nut or a Hindu holy man all week long, and then relaxing a bit on the weekend and having a little feasting. But then every Monday, it's right back to work. Tension/release. Work/rest. There's magic in the ebb and flow.

UNDEREATER'S HABITAT

Undereaters don't have an environment that supports overeating. The cupboards and fridge are not stocked with all types of goodies to forage through.

The house I grew up in, on the other hand, was a playground, a smorgasbord, an amusement park of food. Having all types of stuff available to eat was what made the house a home. That's the way it felt, and that was hard to give up.

A barren house just didn't feel right. It was as if it wasn't really "home" without all the goodies. That had to change. It turns out that home can be very warm, friendly, and loving, even without cookies and chips in the cupboards and ice cream in the freezer.

If you've ever sensed the food in the house "calling" you, you know what food addiction is. There may be a number of foods you cannot have in your house, just like an alcoholic cannot have booze in the house without risking disaster. I've learned that there are a number of foods that I cannot have in my house: cookies, cake, ice cream, chocolate, nuts, and chips top the list. Success is easier without those things around, and

I am not interested in making success any harder than it has to be.

I still eat ice cream and cake, but only on weekends. I'll have it when I'm out, and if I serve it to guests at a party at my place, the leftovers go home with the guests.

Undereaters maintain a "safe" house.

A HEALTH AND FITNESS MENTALITY

People who are fit and trim think differently than the way I thought when I was fat.

I, and my contemporaries, loved the party life. We cherished the most decadent delicacies, and we cherished the lifestyle that celebrated conspicuous consumption. We laughed at the health nuts, and ridiculed their goody two shoes approach to life.

We have to change, and becoming healthy will start by changing the way we think.

We don't have to deny our yen to consume, but we've got to stop celebrating it. Only a fool would champion self-destruction, and we need to stop being fools. So, while we are not bad people to have excessive appetites, we need to stop pretending they are OK. They are not.

We will be well served by beginning to copy some of the beliefs and attitudes of the healthy people.

So, when the party animal in you wants to rave about the delights of the overeating way of life, put it in its place, in the past. Tell it "Quiet!"

Start celebrating health. Start being critical of gluttonous ways of being. Stop approving of unhealthy ways, unhealthy foods, unhealthy pastimes, and unhealthy thinking.

Do this for yourself, for no one else. This is not the same as talking the talk to impress others and then being different when you're by yourself.

We are talking here of a conversion experience. The thinking and behavior that made us fat is one and the same with the obesity itself. We need to stop separating them in our minds. If you hate being fat, start hating the thinking and behavior that made it so.

Becoming an undereater begins by thinking the thoughts of an undereater.

CHAPTER 11

Habituation and Addiction

In the last chapter, I referred to a yen to overeat. We've talked of craving and desire, and in an early chapter, I described conditioning as a process that taps or shapes this force in us: drive, desire.

I have been suggesting you become an undereater, and adopt the behaviors, the habits, and even the thinking of an undereater. How does one become an undereater, one who wants to undereat? The truth is, we want to eat more, sometimes so badly that we can't control ourselves. Isn't it a lie to say we want to think like an undereater, a person who wants to undereat, a person who rejects consuming as a desirable pastime? What about the part of me that just wants to dig in and eat with relish? How can we deny we want to eat?

The question is about desire and the root of desire.

There is a school of thought in Buddhist philosophy that recognizes *attachment* as a central problem, where we become slaves to our attachments (addictions?), unable to let go. The attachments rob us of the freedom to experience happiness, bliss.

When we think of addictions, like heroin addiction or alcoholism, we tend to think that the addiction causes the desire. But this other school of thought proposes that it is the other way around, that the desire causes the attachment. They say that the way to be released from the attachment is to give up the desire.

Easier said than done. How does one become master of desire instead of slave to it? Conditioning certainly plays a role, and we will be looking at more techniques in the coming chapters. But first we need to look a bit more closely at the phenomenon of habit.

My early clinical work focused on alcoholism and substance abuse. In the course of this work, I was surprised to find one clinic for heroin addicts referring to their field as "habit management."

I had always thought of habit management as something they taught in school so you'd get good grades. They encouraged you to have good study habits. Here, they were talking about habit as the most serious of drug addictions.

What is the relation between habit and addiction? Are they the same?

A few chapters back, I spoke of a force being tapped by conditioning to drive us in our behavior, more powerful than your will. Imagine developing habits of undereating, eating fewer calories than you need, so you lose weight, and that these habits become so powerful that they persist on their own, as if you were addicted to them.

Imagine being addicted to undereating instead of being addicted to overeating.

That is precisely what we want to do.

We tend to think that our desires are the real part of us, as true as anything about us, but they are not. Neither are your habits. They are attributes you have taken on, like articles of clothing. They may seem to be the essence of your being, but they are not. Desires and habits are characteristics that you've acquired. As you become more acquainted with the mechanics of your psyche, you'll become more skilled at picking and choosing which ones you want and which ones you don't want. As you become more familiar with the part of you "wearing" these characteristics, and how it works, you will become more able to master desire and habit, rather than be slave to them.

IS HABIT A BLESSING OR A CURSE?

We often think of bad habits when we think of habits, like picking your nose, leaving the seat up, drumming with your fingers, or worse, smoking, eating with your mouth open, stopping at the vending machine every time you pass it, or not flushing.

But you may have many good habits, too: brushing and flossing every morning, closing cabinet drawers and doors, using your turn signals, or checking the gas gauge every time you start the car.

Habits are those routine behaviors we do automatically, without thinking, repetitively, and unconsciously. These behaviors have a life of their own, and are off and running, whether we want them or not. Sometimes they take us to good places, and sometimes they take us in a bad direction.

It's like there is a part of our minds that is on autopilot, like a robotic computer, and these "programs" run on their own, taking us places we may or may not want to be.

Have you ever taken a ride on your day off down a familiar road and found yourself on the way to work instead of going where you intended? You may have started thinking about something else, and then you became aware you were going the wrong way. It's like the car, or your "autopilot," took over, and it ran the "go to work" program or habit.

There is a great deal of mental activity that goes on without our knowledge or will or conscious mind, and it is responsible for the majority of activity we engage in every day. It's called the "subconscious" or "unconscious mind," and it is the realm of habit, among other things. It engages drive without conscious effort, and it gets us through the day easily, making sure our teeth are brushed and we make it to work. It can take us to our dreams.

That is, if we have good habits.

It can also be the path to self-destruction, if the habits we have create a wreck.

Therefore, one of your primary tasks, if you want a happy life, if you want to control your weight, if you want to harness something more powerful than your will to make your dreams come true— is to develop the habits to take you there and kill the habits that wreck you. It's not that hard, but it is not simply a matter of will power. It is work— pure and simple application of effort to a task every day for a while. Then it becomes automatic, a part of you.

The two key elements to habit management are repetition and conditioning.

You may have heard that it takes twenty-one days to create a habit. That's an oversimplification, but the principle is true. Behavior will become habitual simply by doing it enough times every day, by *making* yourself do it for a while, until it starts happening by itself. You actually create neural pathways in your brain by repeating behavior, and after a while, your brain will "run the program" for you, instead of you having to *make* yourself do it. It's like you "wear a path" in your brain, like tramping down the grass in a field, and after a while, a path is worn. Then, when you set out on your hike, you don't have to work so much to get to your destination. The path takes you there. All you have to do is start your day, or your hike, and the habits take you down the path you've worn. The habits happen by themselves. Once established, you no longer have to *make* yourself do them.

If you've ever bought a new car where the levers or ignition was in a new place, you know exactly what I'm talking about. Your hands keep going to the wrong places. There is a force in you, apart from your will, that will help you persist in a task once you have done it a while. We call it "the force of habit."

The first key to habit formation is repetition. Somehow, you get yourself to do the new thing every day for a month, and it will become ingrained, a part of you, a habit.

In the same way, to break a habit, repetition of its absence, or *abstinence*, is key. If you don't use a habit or a path, the weeds start to grow back over, and after a month or so, the habit loses its power. You don't find yourself going down the old trail. You walk the new ones.

Conditioning is the other key. When you want to change habit, make sure you enjoy a reward every time you do the thing you want to develop as a habit. When you want to break a habit, make sure you experience an unpleasant association every time you catch yourself stepping the wrong way. Avoid letting yourself engage in an old, pleasurable bad habit even once, because the rewarding of it will make it more difficult to kill. And we are looking for the easiest way possible to change. We don't want to make it any harder than it has to be.

FOR EXAMPLE

In the last chapter, I talked of copying the behaviors of successful people. One of the key behaviors we want to develop, as a habit, is a daily morning routine or ritual of dreaming of our most heartfelt goals come true. Successful people have a habit of taking a few minutes every morning to do nothing but daydream about how they want their life to be.

In the next chapter, I'll go into more detail about the mental processes I call "Therapeutic Psychogenics," but one of the best uses of them is the daily morning ritual of *imaging* or *visualizing*.

Successful people take a few minutes every morning, perhaps while in the shower or sitting on the john, and they vividly imagine their life as they want it to be. In our case, it would be imagining ourselves at the size and weight we want to be, looking the way we want to look, feeling the way we want to feel, doing the things we want to do.

It is a few moments of reverie, like a meditation. It is the kind of daydreaming that children are so good at, that perhaps you've forgotten how to do in your rush to be a grown up. You are still capable of it, and it will come back quickly if you start doing it again.

Successful people have a habit of doing this every morning, without fail, and the really successful people are dreaming of their life's goals all the time. Let's start with a daily habit of doing it every morning.

When we have gotten to the point of having done it every day for a month, we'll be well on our way to a lifetime habit that would be hard to break. After a month of daydreaming of your dream life every time you sit down on the john, it would be hard *not* to do it every time you sit down. Repetition is key.

To get started, you can use a simple reminder technique of posting a reminder sign, or a picture of your dream, right next to the john or the shower door. Every time you get there, you'll say, "Oh yeah, its time for my imaging exercise." After a month, you'll be hooked.

Conditioning is the other element, and the reinforcement or pleasure here is the excitement and pleasure built into your most heartfelt desires. You must be enough of a kid to have fun daydreaming, and restore your ability to fantasize with gusto. You must be crazy enough to believe in the miracles of life and that all things are possible. Later in the book, we'll address those issues. They are important. You must be willing to let go of cynicism and fear and allow something else to happen, for just a few minutes. Feel the pleasure of the "what if?" thinking. What if you actually got to live the life you'd like?

After a month or so of doing this dreaming exercise every day, you'll have a habit that can lead to all types of new things.

ANOTHER EXAMPLE

Here's an example of killing a habit that took us in the wrong direction and replacing it with a better set.

I was in the habit of eating all night long, pretty much every night. It was a hobby, a pleasant pastime. I'd start with a drink and nuts or something when I got home, and it was pretty much a series of "what's next?" episodes, interrupted by little breaks between snacks. As I said a while back, when I discovered the calories involved in that lifestyle, I realized that there was no way to avoid being obese when one lives that way.

This type of eating habit is an example of one of the toughest of addictions. The spontaneous eating was self-reinforcing with the most primary and powerful of reinforcers, behaviorally. The pleasure of eating, the pleasure principle, the primary experience of libido, of drive and desire satisfied, were all lined up to maintain and strengthen the nighttime eating addiction.

So, first, we need to identify the target behavior, the habits we want to establish.

For me, the meal when I got home at the end of my work day was the most important meal. I often went all day without eating, and didn't think about it much if I was busy. So my food plan was to have small meals at breakfast and lunch, no more than 150 calories each, and have the lion's share of my calories at dinner. I'd plan ahead, and I was thinking about what I'd have on my way home, really looking forward to it.

When I hit the door, I'd pour a glass of Fresca, my favorite drink while fasting, and start preparing dinner. I'd continue fasting while preparing dinner, not nibbling, but fasting. I'd enjoy the sense of achievement and success as I considered that I was burning fat each moment that I fasted, because my body uses energy each moment I'm alive, and I had put next to nothing in it all day. The thoughts of goals achieved and fat burning, because they trigger the experience of deep satisfaction, are pleasures of the highest order, on par with food as a reinforcer, and are powerful tools in habit formation.

I'd have my meal, comprised of my most favorite food in caloric quantities that made me successful, and the pleasure of the food and the success reinforced the habit of eating precisely that way. (As opposed to the diet approach of eating something you really didn't like and then feeling cheated and deprived, or worse, feeling like now, you deserved something good.)

Then, later, when the urge to forage would hit, I'd think to myself, "Wait. I'm fasting and burning fat." That made me feel good, and it served to reinforce the fasting.

I'd think to myself, "If I eat something, which will be overeating, I'll stop burning fat (a loss of something good). Overeating causes the misery and stretch marks and reflux." The association of the negatives with the snacking is called "punishment" in the behavioral sciences and serves to extinguish habit. The more we do this, the less power the old habit has.

When I overcame the urge to overeat, I'd pat myself on the back, and I'd think about the pleasure that my success brings and think about living my life at the weight I wanted to be. Rewarding the victory over the urge to overeat, the decision to wait until the next planned meal, reinforced the fasting behavior and helped to make it a solid habit.

The repetition makes it even stronger. You will get healthier and stronger every time you do this, everyday. The longer you live this way, the easier it gets.

But it is not so easy that you will be invulnerable.

The power of conditioning and habit must be respected.

Clients, when they start finding things surprisingly easy, can get cocky, thinking they are successful because they now have will power. They think they have mastered urges and desire and can now snack with control. "I've got this beaten now," they have said.

The self-reinforcing pleasure of eating has immense power, and unless whatever behavior you contemplate will work as a habit, you need to abstain totally, not even indulging once. It's amazing how something done "just once" can come charging back and take over your life. Your will becomes powerful when you respect the other powers, and it can fade completely away if you defy or deny them.

HABITS TO INSTALL

Clients of The Anderson Method are led to experience months of habit forming technique so that they will be fit for life, so that it will become the new normal for them. It's easier to be led or coached, but there is no reason that you cannot use this information to make big changes in your life right now.

In the last chapter, I revealed some of the habits of undereaters that we can copy. There are programming techniques to install all of them that you can employ. For now, let's identify some of the other habits that are common to people who have been successful with permanent weight control.

GETTING ON THE SCALE FREQUENTLY

The scale and I have had a hate-hate, not a love-hate, relationship, for many years. I still don't love the scale, but I have come to tolerate it and use it to make my life better.

We go way back, and my earliest memories of the scale are of getting weighed in grade school in front of the rest of the class. It was one of the most miserable experiences of my young life, causing many days of non-stop anguish. It amazes me that supposedly bright, educated teachers could engage in this torment. What were they thinking? How could they be so stupid and insensitive?

I didn't go to the doctor for years, and one of the reasons? They weighed you, and it was right out there in a non-private area of the clinic, where there were other people around who could see and hear. It was awful.

Overweight people, even if they don't talk about it, have a problem with being overweight.

Most weight control places weighed you, so I wasn't interested. By the time I was a teen, I'd had enough of being humiliated.

And then, as I became more familiar with the science involved, I began to realize just how stupid and misinformed most of the "experts" were.

I had been led to believe that "the scale doesn't lie," and that the scale is an accurate measure of your progress when you are trying to lose weight. Many people think that behaviorally we need feedback, which is true, and that the scale is a good way to get it, which is *not* true. It turns out that the scale *does* lie, and is about the worst way to measure your progress.

First, remember that to control your weight, you need to develop a lifestyle of habits, where you consume, on average, fewer calories than you burn. You can form a plan and track the calories, and you can know, without any question, whether you won or lost that day. It is fool-proof. The scale cannot measure that.

Behaviorally, calorie tracking is perfect because you will know, beyond any doubt, where you stand. You can feel confident and successful, and you will reinforce precisely the behavior that needs to be reinforced, eating the foods you like in a way that keeps you from being fat.

The scale, on the other hand, is just as likely to go up on a day you undereat as it is to go down. It measures mainly the water in your body. If you believe the scale measures your progress, you are likely, when you are retaining fluids, to feel like a failure on a day you succeed. You'll end up punishing and extinguishing the behavior that needs to be reinforced, and you'll make a mess of any attempts to form good habits.

If you overeat and indulge in obesity-producing behavior, but get a bit dehydrated, the scale will go down. If you believe in it, you'll think the overeating is OK, and you'll be programming in obesity-producing habits! It's a prescription for failure.

The scale, on a day-to-day, week-to-week, and even month-to-month basis, will never honestly measure your progress when you are trying to lose weight.

The scale measures all the matter that's contained within your skin: fat, muscle, bone, organs, blood, the contents of your bladder and bowel. Your body is about seventy percent water, so it measures mainly the water.

Your body can have a range of as much as ten pounds on the scale between when you are dehydrated, like when you have spent all day in the sun without anything to drink, and when you are retaining fluids, like after a weekend where you had Chinese food, a ham dinner, spicy foods, and sugary desserts.

There is no way the scale will give you accurate feedback on the results of your efforts. You could have a wonderfully successful day, and the scale may go up. You could have a great week, where you lose a pound or two of fat, and the scale may go up. If you thought the scale was an accurate measure, you'd feel hopeless.

Imagine going a month without weighing, because you were told that weighing once a month was a way to avoid being discouraged, a sure way to feel accomplished. They tell you to weigh only once a month, and you are sure to be happy with it.

You could have a tremendously successful month, losing as much as ten pounds of fat, if we could isolate and measure it. After a month of working hard, eating right, working out, losing ten pounds of fat, gaining muscle, getting healthier, imagine that you get on the scale and "gain" a few pounds, because you got more fit and happen to be retaining fluid that day! All that work— and for nothing! If you believed in the scale as the measure of your success, you'd feel like jumping off a bridge. The scale lies. Don't believe it.

How about the people who indulge in their food addiction, and then take diuretics before the "weigh-in?" They drop a few pounds and are applauded! Behaviorally, guess what happens? They reward overeating, taking diuretics, and peeing all day. Those are the desires and habits they are installing!

Forget about trusting the scale. It is a liar. It will never help you lose weight. In fact, it interferes when it won't consistently reward your successful efforts.

If all we were interested in was losing the weight, we'd be better off without the scale. Just track the calories, and you'll know every day you've won. You will burn off a bit of fat every day, and you'll feel successful every day.

So, why is getting on the scale all the time a good idea?

It helps to maintain the weight loss once you've taken it off.

Getting on the scale every day for the rest of your life will help you to stay successful.

You'll see it move within a range that you'll become familiar with, the high when you are retaining fluid, and the low when you get dehydrated. You get on the scale every day, and as long as you are within your range, you are doing a good job with your maintenance eating. But, the day you see it move above the high end of your range, alarms go off, and you return to the low calories you need to hit to lose weight. You stay with your real low undereating until the scale shows you that you can hit the low end of your range.

With The Anderson Method, we get on the scale every day, and we keep a chart, but we record only the lows. While we are eating in a way to lose weight, we get on it every day, looking to see if we will hit a new low today. If it does, it feels great, and we write it down. If it stays the same or goes up, we call it a liar, and look to our calorie tracking to give us a pat on the back. And we look forward to the day when it will go down again, and we can enter a new low. It will come, guaranteed, when we are undereating.

People who are successful at weight control get on the scale every day. They are very conscious of where they are on the scale. It is a part of their everyday life and consciousness. But it is not their god, and it frequently is a liar.

INFREQUENT FESTIVITY

In the last chapter, I introduced the idea of eating real austere during the week and then relaxing and eating more on the weekend.

Fit people indulge in festivity every once in a while, but not all the time.

Some of us got the notion that it was a good idea to have the "good life" all the time. Thanksgiving was pretty good, so why not have it every day? Those great restaurant meals they advertise are really great, so why not have a feast every day, at every meal?

Why? Because it will kill you. You can't be healthy and feast and party all the time. Once in a while is OK, but not all the time.

So, healthy successful people have habits where they don't eat out and go to parties every day. They don't have luncheon parties during the week. Most don't eat lunch out at all, except low-calorie fast food selections. Most fix their own lunches or use shakes or low-calorie frozen microwave meals. Most don't go out or go to parties during the week. They are festive infrequently and stay pretty low key and austere most of the time.

I live in an area where many people have been able to retire in style, and they have looked forward to it, sometimes thinking that they should be able to live like they were on permanent vacation, living the high life every day. Many end up gaining lots of weight, and when they find out that the price of that lifestyle is obesity and all the problems that come with it, they are mad. They feel like they have been cheated.

If you've had an idea in the back of your mind that some day you should be able to just indulge without keeping a lid on it, forget it. We will, for the rest of our lives, need to work at our health and well being. It can be wonderful, pleasurable work, but there is no retirement from responsibility. You can indulge in festivity occasionally, but most of the time we need to be austere.

Healthy people indulge in festivities infrequently.

SPEED SHOPPING WITH A LIST

I talked earlier about managing the environment at home, making your home a "safe house." With The Anderson Method, we generalize that principle to take into account all environments where we are presented with eating cues— stimuli, in the language of behaviorism.

Successful people never go into a grocery store without a list, and they buy only what's on the list. They don't wander around and look at all the work the merchants have done to get them to buy things, as if we needed anything more compelling than the sight and smells of the foods we enjoy.

I was such a sucker when I was in stores that I developed a technique of "speed shopping" to avoid impulse buying. I play a game where I try to see how fast I can get all the things on my list and get out. I try to see if I can make it all the way through the store without stopping, grabbing the items off the shelves as I pass.

I've been asked "How do you check the prices? Don't you end up paying too much and missing the sale items?"

My priority is succeeding at controlling my weight, and everything else takes a back seat to that. If it costs more to succeed, that's OK with me. Besides, the marketplace forces keep things from getting too out of line. I trust that my fellow shoppers will keep the merchants somewhat in line, price-wise. With what you've probably paid to lose weight in the past, and what you'd be willing to pay for something that really works, if you're like most of us, the cost of speed shopping is nothing. Look at the time you'll save!

KEEP YOUR EYES AND EARS OPEN FOR IDEAS

There is no limit to the behaviors we could list that would help us to be successful if we made them our habits.

Magazines and popular media will forever be telling stories of tips and "how tos" related to weight loss, and every once in a while, you'll come across an idea you want to use. Everyone is different, so some will fit your personality and some won't. Try things. Some things you'll want to make habits, and you'll know how to use the tools of conditioning and repetition or persistence to build your repertoire of success habits.

On the other hand, you have some bad habits that have been a curse instead of a blessing.

You know that some of the things that you do habitually need to die off for you to be successful. You're aware of some of them already, and you'll become aware of more as you read on. You will need to work hard in applying the mechanics of conditioning to kill those bad habits. If you are able to decide you want to stop them, and decide to use the "brainwashing" tools to kill them off, you can be successful, with persistence. Once begun, repetition will be on your side. If you begin now, months from now, you will be surprised that you used to do some of the things that seem unchangeable now.

We are creatures of habit. We are born predisposed to addiction. And the sooner we recognize this and decide what to do with it, the better off we will be.

We will have habits. That's the way we're made. We have no choice in that. We *do* have a choice in what habits to have. We will be addicted to one thing or another, attached to something as long as we live. We have the power to make it something that is healthy or unhealthy. Let's kill the unhealthy habits and addictions, and get addicted to what makes us healthy and whole— truly happy, not just stimulated with intoxicating pleasures. We need to extinguish the addictions that are killing us. The way to do that is to become addicted to the healthy things.

CHAPTER 12

Therapeutic Psychogenics

What are the roots of desire? How do we get motivated to make our wishes and dreams become reality? Can we create an inner impulse to initiate the action needed to accomplish our goals? Is there a way to make ourselves *feel* like doing what's good for us instead of what's not? Can we get ourselves to *want* to do what's good for us, instead of feeling like we have to, but don't want to? Is there a way to enhance the power to change our habits and addictions, change ourselves, in addition to conditioning?

Yes.

And it's not just gritting your teeth and trying to use will power.

In order to make the changes you'll need, there are a few prerequisites that you will need to contribute that we'll go over later; for now, I want to make you familiar with some of the most important elements of The Anderson Method that I call "Therapeutic Psychogenics." These elements are largely responsible for the miraculous sounding changes that clients report when they say that they are able to do things that had always been impossible for them, sometimes saying that succeeding has been easy, when it was never even possible before.

Psychogenics refers to the phenomena where mental and physical states or conditions are developed as a result of conscious or unconscious psychological forces or processes. Mostly, the word is used when we talk of *disorders* that are caused by the mind. Think of disorders where the disease has its origin, not with physical causes, like germs, virus, or toxins, but with the mental processes of the sufferer.

The mind can create all types of illness, and this has been known in medicine for many years. For years now, cases of blindness and paralysis have been documented to be caused, not by physical disease or trauma, but by psychological trauma. We are not talking of the problem being imaginary or "all in their head," as if it wasn't real. The blindness or paralysis is very real, but manufactured by the mind of the sufferer, in the same way that vision or locomotion is manufactured by the mind. The brain creates the experience of the patient, and it is very real. The blindness or inability to move is no less real than the ability to see or move. It is not that the patient wants or is able to control the problem, or is even conscious of the process. Often, it is totally unconscious factors that cause the condition, and it is totally contrary to the patient's wishes or will. It is disorder entirely generated by unconscious mental processes.

You may think that in these cases, the body doesn't really change, but psychological forces actually do change physical conditions. We know that many conditions, like hives and rashes, and stomach and digestive problems, are often caused by our mental processes. Panic attacks, where the body races out of control, with tachycardia, hyperventilation, nausea and vomiting, are examples of the body's disorder being generated entirely by the mind. High blood pressure, immune dysfunction, diabetes, heart disease, and chronic pain have all been linked to psychological forces.

Over the years, we have been discovering not only the mind's ability to create illness, but to cure it.

It is very interesting to observe that placebos, the sugar pills that are used in experiments to compare to drugs being tested, often get good results in curing illness! Those taking pills that they *think* might cure them, often *do* get better, and in greater numbers than the people not taking anything.

It seems that when a person *expects* that they will get better, the mind and brain do something to make it happen.

This is a good example of what I call "Therapeutic Psychogenics," psychological processes, conscious or unconscious, that generate the healing or curing of disorders that generate healthy conditions, health, in the body.

There are many cases on record of spontaneous unexplainable recoveries, from all types of disorders, where miraculous healing seems to take place. The recovery, thought to be impossible or possible only with extraordinary medical intervention, has been explained as the result of faith, prayer, or God's will. We know that the body has the ability to heal. Some say that the person's extraordinary belief is what summons the body's healing power. They say that the person's belief and expectation is what gives the brain the correct directions to do its work, to send the right messages to all the systems, to heal the body. I believe this to be true, and explaining it as such makes it no less miraculous or divine.

Today, hospital patients are led to meditate and engage in hypnosis-like exercises where they tell their body to heal, where they imagine tumors shrinking and bad cells being killed and eaten by the good cells. We know that when a person does this, the brain sends out messages to all the organs, through the nervous system, contacting every structure in the body and sending messages to be well. We know that the body has the systems to heal itself and function properly, and it is thought that the way to have the brain operate those systems is to vividly imagine it.

Hypnosis, placebos, positive thinking, prayer— these are all examples of what I term "Therapeutic Psychogenics," the engaging of conscious and unconscious psychological forces to cure and heal us.

We know today that your brain takes its direction from your thoughts and your imagination, and it will work to create what you think about, what you imagine. If you were a client in therapy, we have an exercise where we can demonstrate this to you in an instant, so that there will never again be any doubt whatsoever of that fact. But just wanting or willing something is not enough. The factors that contribute to the conscious and unconscious psychological forces are complex and not entirely knowable. So, there are a number of principles, techniques, practices, and habits that are helpful to respect when deciding to lose weight for good, or to make any changes, for that matter.

The *visualization* or *imaging* technique that we discussed earlier is one of the most important of the Therapeutic Psychogenics, but there are many.

SELF IMAGE AND BODY IMAGE

At one time, I had a great deal of difficulty believing I could be anything but three hundred pounds. I was told I needed to develop a fit body image, but it was impossible. I couldn't even imagine it. Being fit was something the other people did. It just wasn't in my nature. That's the way I thought at the time.

As long as we allow this kind of belief system to remain, we will be fighting powers greater than our will in trying to make a change. Something inside us will be working twenty-four/seven to keep us the way we have been.

The idea is that our brain and unconscious mind, that which controls everything in our body and activities, takes its orders from our imagination and thoughts. It controls our immune system, all our organs, our appetites and desire, our metabolism, and our habits, among other things.

If we're sick, and we imagine ourselves getting better, the mind and brain know what to do to make us better, and they send out the messages to all our systems to do the job to make us get better. Our unconscious mind also controls our habits and desires. It runs the programs to help us get better and makes us feel like doing what it takes to get better.

Unfortunately, if we imagine ourselves getting sicker, it knows what to do to make that happen, too, and is likely to send out the messages to make things unhealthy.

If we imagine ourselves as someone who is three hundred pounds, it knows how to do that, too, and it sends out the messages to make that happen. It will send out messages so that programs will run to keep us three hundred: the habits, the desires, the impulses, the appetites, and perhaps even the metabolic rate, to make someone three hundred pounds; all those mental "programs" would be turned on to make us stay three hundred pounds.

That's why, when we are trying to lose weight, we are encouraged to think of ourselves as being successful, losing weight, hitting our goal weight, and doing all the things we'd like to do when we are the weight we want to be. The idea is that the brain will send out the messages to make that happen. The unconscious mind will turn on and run the habits to make us lose weight; it will have us feeling the desire to do what it takes to lose weight, and will make everything in us, our appetites, our motivation, even our body systems, conspire to make us lose weight.

This will only happen if we believe it's possible, because we imagine what we believe, unconsciously, twenty-four/seven. We might be led by a diet coach to think about losing weight for a moment and get excited and motivated, but if we really believe it can't be done, we'll go back to imagining ourselves fat, twenty-four/seven, and the brain knows exactly what to do to make that happen. We'd be back on the fat program, twenty-four/seven.

So, belief is key. Our thoughts and imaginings are the things that bring reality into being, that tell our brain and unconscious mind what to do, *but our beliefs are the thoughts and imaginings we have running non-stop, twenty-four/seven,* even in our sleep. Beliefs have even more power than habits of thought. Belief can *create* habits of thought.

What do you believe about yourself? What do you believe yourself to be?

This is why self-image, self-concept, and body image are so critical: You will be working twenty-four/seven, unconsciously, to become what you believe yourself to be. If you believe you are weak-willed with no self-control, your mind knows how to make that happen. If you believe you are destined to be fat, because the whole family is like that, your mind will be working twenty-four/seven to make you that way, too. If, when you think of yourself, you can't imagine anything but a fat body, your mind knows exactly what to do to make it real, and you'll have the habits, appetites, and desires to make it so.

When I was overweight, I thought I'd get the weight off first, and then I'd be able to think of myself as successful and fit. But I was never able to be successful until I started believing and imagining it happening. I had to first develop the belief that I could be successful, that I could be a thin person. While I was a wreck, I had to start by believing I could be different, and I wasn't *made* to be a wreck. While I was three hundred pounds, I had to first be able to imagine myself thinner. I had to believe I was made to be healthy instead of a wreck. When I started to imagine and believe these new things, only then was I able to make them happen.

What is your self-concept? Are you your body, or are you the person who inhabits that body? Are you a collection of habits and conditions, or are you the person who has them, who wears them? Is your ill health a mistake to be corrected, or is it the way nature or God intends things to be?

You will be able to change the conditions, the body and the habits, if you see that you are the person or "soul" at the center, the one who wears them, rather than the conditions themselves. If you think that the habits you have and the fat body are the "real" you, you are stuck. If you believe our unhealthy ways are the way nature or God made things to be, instead of a mistake of our own doing that needs to be corrected, you are stuck.

When we are born, we are not even conscious of what we are. It takes a while to figure out that our sense and control seems to stop at the bounds of our skin, limited to our body. That's when we start to establish our consciousness and self concept. And then we start to develop beliefs about ourselves, based on our models, our parents, our world, and what they tell us. We then start to create our "self," based on our beliefs about ourselves, and what seems to be true. We have often been wrong. I know I was. You know that you have been wrong about things in the past, and you are probably not right all the time, even now.

To succeed, we need to let go of some old mistaken beliefs and adopt some healthier ones: that you are not your body or your habits; that they are no more your true nature than your haircut or your overcoat; that you are a being or soul whose nature, like all life, is to flourish; that you were made to be healthy and fit, like all the other creatures running around, like the squirrels and deer. It is not natural for them to be obese, and it is not your true nature either. We made a mistake, and we can correct it. We need to start believing that our true self, if it were to emerge, is fit and healthy, full of vitality and a tendency to health. We need to imagine ourselves healthy.

When you think of yourself, if you cannot imagine yourself thin, as it was with me, you need to create a fit image that will allow you to imagine what you'll look like when you remove the overcoat of fat you've acquired. Get a photo of your head, make a copy, and trim it down so you see your face looking out from a different shape, with the cheeks and chin reformed. Use a copier to copy a photo, blown-up, and cut a well-shaped head from it. Then, look through the clothing ads for a body shape you'd like and copy that. Recopy your cut-out head and get the size right by using the zoom feature so it's the right proportion to the body. Lastly, paste your head on the body and copy it again, adjusting the darkness until it looks OK.

With a little work, you will be able to create a picture that looks the way you'll look when you lose the excess weight. Then you'll be able to imagine what you look like when the mistake is corrected, when you are at the weight you were really meant to be. When I first saw this picture, something happened inside me, and I see the same thing happen with all my clients who had trouble imagining themselves fit. Something changes. Something stirs. It makes it possible for us to imagine ourselves fit. Being able to visualize what we want has power.

The single most powerful item in your toolbox of Therapeutic Psychogenics is your self-concept, including your body image. Your old self-concept is a habit. You've thought it over and over again so much that you might believe it. But, you can change. You start by deciding to believe in what is really true and right, not because it's what you grew up with, but because you can. You can look at the healthier, happier you, and you can make it a habit until it is more familiar, more true, than the old you.

MODELING

When we are born, there are two main ways we acquire behavior, or learn. One is conditioning. If something feels good, our computer-like brain locks in on the behavior, and we acquire it, or learn it. We also have the automatic tendency to repeat it, and we experience desire or motivation to do it again and again.

The other main mechanism is modeling. We take in information from our environment, including the sights and sounds of others, and copy the behavior. Doing this is the way we are made. It is not something we want to do or choose to do. It is the way our mind/body works. We can simply see someone do something, and our natural tendency is to copy it. Our eyes see something; our mind constructs a mental model of it; and then it produces a copy.

If you have ever heard yourself say something, and then been aghast that it sounded like one of your parents, you realize that this copying is neither chosen, nor conscious, nor desired. It is the way you are made. There is something in you that will make you automatically work to create a reality of the models in your mind. It triggers drive and motivation without any act on your part, other than to observe.

Now, armed with this information, you can consciously decide to stop copying role models you'd rather not follow and intentionally choose some who are trailblazing the path you'd like to take. It, like self-concept and all the other examples of Therapeutic Psychogenics we'll look at, reaches in and taps that power in you where drive, desire, motivation, and habit come from. When you align your will with that, you'll start getting somewhere. Start thinking about the models in your life.

For me, this meant considering my entire family of parents, grandparents, aunts, and uncles, and deciding I was *not* just like my father's side (which I had always been told). I needed better models, and I needed to enthusiastically embrace them, something you may not be prone to do as a "mature grown-up."

Children are great examples of modelers, and it's easy to spot them picking up the language, attitudes, lifestyles, and behaviors of their heroes and those they hang out with. It works like magic. We need to be enthusiastic modelers, like children, but only with healthy models.

We are not destined or fated to be like those we have modeled in the past. All we need to do is look around and pick out new models. It can become a pastime to keep your eyes open and take note of those in your world whom you will definitely *not* follow and those who are showing you precisely how you'd *like* to live. When you think of them, make your intentions clear. It's not like you have to consciously work at mimicking them. Just decide which ones you'll follow. Once you've selected them, it works on its own, unconsciously.

You can begin putting the power of this phenomenon to work today as you realize how you may have unconsciously used this badly, when you thought of others who have made wrecks of their lives. When you've seen the wrecks and thought "I hope that's not my future," you were mistakenly giving your brain an unhealthy pattern to follow when you imagined yourself like them. Stop doing that.

Thank God for those who have lived well and shown us how it's done. Pick out some new heroes. Put their pictures up in your place. Imagine yourself like your heroes. It's not just for teenagers.

WRITTEN GOALS

Something very powerful happens when you write goals down. You involve a number of senses and mental processes, and focus your mind, and you suggest to yourself that this thing is going to happen. It's a very effective form of self-hypnosis.

Some people read their goals every day, and some re-write them frequently. There are countless people who will testify to the power of writing down your goals, with stories that border on the mystical. I am among them.

The power of this technique can be employed with something as simple as a "to do" list, a letter, a diary entry, or a sign on your bathroom mirror saying "120 by May 1."

It took me a long time to warm up to the idea of goals. When I was a kid, and the grown ups would push them on me, it always had to do with what they wanted, not I, and there was always the trap of getting judged and not being good enough. I learned to hate the idea of goals. But I have a new take on the subject now.

The written goals I'm speaking of have nothing to do with anyone else. It's simply taking the step of admitting to yourself what you'd really like. You don't have to share these ideas with anyone. Just let yourself admit to yourself what you'd really like, if it was possible.

Written goals have made miracles for me, but I don't think one of them has ever happened precisely as I had planned. I had to consistently crumple up paper and reconfigure the goals that hadn't happened as I wished, which was pretty much all of them, but something kept me moving in the right direction.

Remember, these are techniques to program the unconscious to do the work for you. Your part is to identify and enter the goal into the computer. When you first admit what goals you'd like, don't worry so much about how to get there, or having to perform. It's not a contest. It's just a more concrete form of the dreaming and imagining I spoke of earlier.

CYBERNETICS

The word "cybernetics" describes the discipline of comparing the human control mechanism, the brain, to mechanical control mechanisms, computers, to develop an understanding of the way our brain works, and perhaps ways we can make it better.

They are both electronic devices that channel the flow of current in order to execute action of some sort. A muscle or lever is moved, a sound is made, an emotion or desire is felt.

We tend to think we should be able to just decide, with our will, what should happen, but we know that doesn't always work. On the other hand, when we are confronted with things like habits, addictions, desire, and cravings that seem to have a life of their own, often contrary to our will, we are at a loss to explain them or control them.

Both traditional psychologies and cybernetics observe that human beings are goal-oriented, goal-seeking creatures. We are continuously engaged in behavior that seeks to satisfy some need, want, or desire. It goes on even in our sleep.

Cybernetics compares this to the goal-attaining behavior of computers, which are given instructions of what to do, what programs to run, through a keyboard, and asks, "How does the brain get it's instructions of what programs to run and what to seek?"

If the brain is a computer that does all this conscious and unconscious stuff, how do we type in the instructions so that it does what we want and takes us where we want to go, rather than some other direction?

VISION POSTING OR VISION MAPPING

The psychologists who took this cybernetic approach are largely responsible for all the attention that visualization and imaging have gotten. They have given us a logical way to understand how the brain is programmed. The act of writing out your goal is a way of typing into the computer what you want it to do, and imagining it is precisely how we "power" up the brain to produce it for us.

Picturing something, imagining it, thinking about it, is the equivalent of typing in the destination for a computer-operated robot and pushing the button "enter."

Years ago, mystics of one form or another told us to imagine and pray and believe and that a mysterious power, beyond our will, would deliver. Now, the psychologists give us an explanation of the phenomenon, even if they can't explain what its origin or real mechanism is.

What they say has tremendous value. For a generation prone to believe in science and doubt the mystics, we now have a startling reason to pay attention to what we think about and what we imagine. We know how effective computers can be, and we hear that the brain is the most complex computer in existence.

Thinking about and imagining something, not "just" using will power, is the way to set everything within us to work on creating that thing. It brings all the powers within us to bear on the task, not the least of which is desire and habit.

If we were careless with what we thought and imagined before, we now have a scientific reason to pay attention. If we imagine something nasty, what we don't want, what we fear, we are stupidly putting the most powerful computer the world has ever seen on the task of creating what we don't want.

We need to pay attention to what we imagine and think about.

For those of us who desperately want some heartfelt desire, like losing weight and staying at our ideal weight forever, we have the secret: imagine it. Think about it and visualize it all the time. Believe it is the way you were made to be, and see it happening.

This is why the daily habit of spending a few moments every day imagining yourself at your goal is so powerful. You are, in that simple act, putting the world's most powerful computer on the job to get you what you want most in the world.

This is why we dream of it vividly, and why we want to feel the excitement and pleasure it will bring. The stimulation of emotion and visual senses increases the brain cells and synapses involved.

This is why we write our goals down. We are involving the sense of touch when we write, the verbal part of our brain when we think in words, and the visual part of our brain when we think in pictures, as well as seeing the "command" we have written down. Writing out our goals is the act of very effectively programming our supercomputer, making sure it gets the instructions right.

Which brings us to vision posting, or vision mapping.

This is an incredibly simple tool, deceptively simple, yet more powerful in some ways than all the rest.

Vision posting, or vision mapping, is the simple act of posting in your environment the images of your life's vision. You can post pictures, and you can post words. You post in your house, your office, or your car, the pictures and descriptions of what you want in your life. What you want your life to be like, and what you want to have and be, should be posted. Whatever your goals are, you post the pictures and words that cause your brain to see it, think it, vividly, to construct the model in your mind as it takes in the information.

In our case we post pictures of us at the weight we want to be. We post pictures of the beach, or parties, or tennis— all with the images of you enjoying life at the weight you want to be. We post signs that say, "I win and feel good every day I undereat." "I am becoming 120 pounds, for life." "140 this summer."

The beauty of the posting is that once you've put the pictures and signs up, they work on their own. You don't have to decide to do anything, as you do with the morning ritual. Every time you walk by them, the eyes see them, like cameras delivering the info to the computer, and the information is processed, even if you're not aware of it. It's automatic.

Remember, with all of these practices, the idea is to program your supercomputer to do it for you, rather than just try to use will power. We want to program the brain, which has charge of all the programs (the habits, desires, craving, and motivation) to work on taking you where you want to go. Instead of fighting you, your unconscious supercomputer will be helping you.

WHO ELSE IS PROGRAMMING YOU?

Make sure you pay attention to what else is being posted for your brain to imagine. If you are watching TV or passing a billboard, you just might process the wrong goal. You have the world's best computer at your disposal, and if you give it a donut or potato chips to imagine, don't be surprised if a program starts running to motivate you in the wrong direction. We'll talk more about this.

STIMULUS CONTROL

We've discussed having a safe house without the foods that you can't control, and racing through the grocery store to avoid being tempted by things you've had a weakness for. We've also talked about changing the media you pump through your brain. Here's the reason why it's so important, and another example of how unconscious processes can have such an impact on your life: Pavlovian or "classical" conditioning.

Pavlov was a scientist who made a great contribution to the understanding of our mental operations with his now famous experiment. He rang a bell every time he fed his dog, and after a while, when the bell rang, the dog would salivate, even though there was no food present.

A condition was created where the brain would operate the salivary glands, as if the dog was eating, even though the dog wasn't eating.

We learned we could push the "eat" button in the brain just by ringing the bell. This triggering of the salivary gland is a more significant piece of information than your pet coming when you use the can opener.

You may think that the can opener makes your dog or cat think there's something to eat, but Pavlov's experiment shows there is something much more remarkable going on.

People, and dogs, too, don't and can't salivate because they decide to. Try it. You can't just decide to salivate. Those glands are operated by a system that functions below your level of consciousness, and they are turned on or off automatically and are normally beyond your ability to control. The only way you can make your salivary glands pump is to eat, or think of eating, which is the equivalent of ringing the bell.

This shows us a way to control some of the unconscious processes that you may have believed were uncontrollable.

There are a number of unconscious automatic responses that you have, such as desires and cravings, that have not been within your power to control, or so you thought. It turns out that many of them have been triggered by stimulus, like the bell, that you didn't pay much attention to. Various things in your environment have been pushing buttons in your brain, and creating lots of urges, desires, and cravings. Fighting them has been a lot of work for you, trying to control yourself. Wouldn't life be so much easier if you could eliminate half, or more, of the urges you get?

Recovering alcoholics who want to avoid a relapse identify the "triggers" or "cues" that lead them to thoughts of drinking and learn to avoid them or develop strategies to negate them. That's what we need to do.

There are probably hundreds of things that trigger the thoughts desires and urges you get, and you'll have to start paying attention, so you can cut down on the number of times you'll need to manage it. If the "bell" doesn't ring, there is no drooling or urges and cravings to deal with.

What are your "bells?" Do you do OK until you pass the vending machine? Find a new route to take.

Does your mouth start watering as soon as you get off work, because you've had a treat when you got home every day for years? Better change to that technique I use. Start a diet drink as soon as you get home, and then start preparing what you're going to eat, and then eat it. If you get off at three, like a teacher, find a new activity to engage in after work. Go to the gym or walk the beach, instead of snacking and watching TV.

When I was younger, just passing the fridge or the kitchen would trigger an urge, and I'd be opening doors. Living without a kitchen would be one option, but not very realistic. I have no food in the house that's not part of the meals I've planned on. There is no food that's for spontaneous eating. It took a while to stop having urges when I passed the kitchen, but with nothing to eat as a snack, it died out after a while.

I found that if certain foods found there way into the house, just having them there, or knowing they were there, would cause urges to happen. If I got rid of the snacks, there was no problem. If they were there, they would "call" me continuously, until they were gone. Now, that stuff goes home with the guests, or it gets tossed when I wash the dishes. For me, no nuts, chips, cookies, cakes, ice cream, chocolate candy, or wine in the house. I've tried to eat them in a controlled fashion, and I can't. I'll just keep going back for "a bit more" until it's gone. I only have those things when I'm dining out, or entertaining guests who will take the leftovers with them.

There may be dishes that you are in the habit of nibbling on while you prepare them. I can't make potato salad without sampling a bit in the process of making it. I failed at trying to make it without the sampling (which can easily add up to hundreds of calories). Potato salad is no longer a regular item on my menu. I make it perhaps once a year, on a weekend. And, oh yes, it doesn't stay in the house. It's one of those things that will "call" me if it's in the house.

You may need to drive home by a different route; quit bowling; quit bridge; quit coffee hour at church. You may even need to stop keeping company with some people.

Pay attention to the stimuli in your life, the "bells" that cause your urges and desires to pop up. You will always have urges, and you'll need to deal with them in an effective way, but life will be easier the fewer you have. Pay attention when you get an urge and see if you can identify the trigger or cue. Then decide if it is something you want to change. You *can* have an effect on the urges. They are not beyond your control.

AVERSIVE CONDITIONING

You can't eliminate all the urges. They will happen for the rest of your life. It's good to reduce the number you have to deal with, but you must develop a way to meet them and beat them when you have them.

"Covert sensitization" is the technical term for one of the "brainwashing" techniques that clients find most useful. I described it before when I talked about imagining maggots in the jelly donuts.

When you get an urge, there is a two-step process to meet it and beat it. When you catch yourself considering eating something, you don't have to think about it and decide if it will fit in your diet plan. It won't. Remember, you'll be fasting until your next planned meal. There is no need to decide whether something is OK or not. It's not. It's overeating if it is not part of the meal you've planned.

So first, you talk to yourself— out loud, if you're alone. "Wait. That would be overeating, which causes the fat and stretch marks I hate. I'm on my way to 120, and I'm going to love going to the beach. I'm *so* looking forward to buying a size smaller."

Then you picture or think of whatever you were thinking of eating in a disgusting or unappetizing way. Imagine that the people who handled it didn't wash their hands after using the bathroom. Imagine that the food's infested with bugs. When you catch yourself feeling like eating some unplanned thing, intervene and link it with something unpleasant, and it will change the way you feel. Do it enough, and it will permanently change the way you feel about that food. You'll not only fight off that urge, but you'll be reprogramming the unconscious part of your mind that runs the desire and habit programs. You'll have fewer urges in the future to deal with. It really is brainwashing.

SELF-TALK

When I described cognitive behavior therapy, I said that we may not be aware of it, but we all have a constant monologue going on in our heads, below the level of consciousness. This unconscious thought world can be influenced and changed if it has been causing problems.

I described how powerful beliefs are, and I pointed out that we often have irrational beliefs that mess things up. The belief that the scale proves you failed if it goes up a pound when you drink a glass of water is a good example.

Intellectually, you may understand that holding a glass of water when you step on the scale does not mean that you did not succeed that day. You may know that you had to burn some fat if you ate only one thousand calories. But still, when you step on the scale and it goes up, there will be a part of you that believes you failed, that *feels* that way. This happens because there is a monologue going on, that you may or may not be aware of, that says, "I'm gaining weight even though I ate the right way. This is hopeless. I might as well eat whatever I feel like." If we allow this to go on, it will have a powerful effect.

Instead, we've got to be saying, "I know I burned fat today, because of the calories I ate. This must be water weight that will change tomorrow. Maybe tomorrow the scale will hit a new low." Even if you doubt it's true, say it. Say it enough, and it will start to feel true. You'll begin to believe it.

Real brainwashers have known for years that they can get you to act and feel like something is true, even if you intellectually know it's false, simply by repeating the lie over and over again. They simply say it repeatedly, and the unconscious part of your mind will accept it as true if you haven't been labeling it a lie in your self-talk. Advertisers and propagandists are betting that if they say something often enough, the unconscious part of your mind will start acting and feeling like it's true. They are more interested in working with that part of your mind, anyway. They show young, beautiful, sexy, athletic people with cigarettes, and there is a part of your brain that feels like smoking and health go together. You will then act and feel like it's OK to do something that you know causes cancer. They do the same thing with calorie-laden food. They show healthy, active people eating in a gluttonous way, and there is a part of you that feels like that lifestyle is OK.

Hear something enough, or tell it to yourself enough, and you will come to believe it.

So, start paying attention to ads, and yell "Liars!" when you see those ads. Point out how ridiculous they are, how insulting, how harmful. Don't listen to lying politicians without pointing out the lies. The way to prevent the lies from having an influence is to be aware of them and refute them. That will stop the negative brainwashing.

Take charge of what you hear, and what goes in your mind, by writing the script yourself. Start paying attention to your self-talk, and say the things you want to be true in your life. Stop saying things like "I gain weight no matter what I do." Start saying things like "I am becoming 120 by undereating every day. I know I'm winning every day because I undereat and know my calories."

Never say "I don't care." You know you do, but if you say that kind of thing, a part of you will believe it and act as if it were true. Don't say things that would ruin your life if they came to pass. Your self-talk has power.

SELF-HYPNOSIS

"Self-hypnosis" refers to the phenomenon of making auto-suggestions, like "I am succeeding at this," and then, simply by doing that, your mind goes to work on it and makes it happen.

It is not hocus-pocus or anything you need to learn how to do. You've been doing it all your life. But maybe not in a good way. You may have been using it to ruin things if you've said things like "No matter what I do, I gain it back."

Unconsciously responding to suggestion is simply the way we are made. If someone says, "look," it takes an almost superhuman effort not to. You automatically and unconsciously act to do what you're told, and what's been forecast.

Most people think that hypnosis is some magical kind of thing where a command is said once, and then "poof!" Everything is different. There are some powerful ways, involving altered states of consciousness that are quite remarkable, but there is no hypnosis that is as powerful as the suggestions you make to yourself everyday, all day long.

Good self-hypnosis would involve you saying every morning, "I'm getting better at this undereating every day. It's not even hard anymore. I'm losing weight like crazy."

Bad self-hypnosis would be saying, "This will never work. I'll never change."

I've seen clients use both, and I've seen both work.

When you start paying attention to your self-talk, imagine that it is a Svengali, a proven mind controller, who is saying these things, and they cause you to make them happen, like a zombie in a trance. In that case, only a fool would allow all those self-destructive things to be said. Don't be a fool. Don't utter any forecasts that aren't something you would pray for. Don't affirm something you'd rather were not true.

In truth, there is a Svengali whispering in your ear all the time. It is you.

SUGGESTION

Not only do we need to become more aware of our self-talk, but we need to pay more attention to the unspoken messages we respond to.

When you are given a plate of food, no one says that this amount is appropriate and you should eat this much, but when you are given the dish, the action has an unspoken message: Eat this. If you were lost in conversation, you may later realize that you ate something you had no intention of eating, and you weren't even aware of it until after you finished.

If you have serving dishes, family style, on the table, the unspoken message here is "eat more." And like zombies in a trance, we often do, without a thought.

If you refrain from putting serving dishes on the table, you'll find it much easier to eat only the portions you planned on. You won't feel as much desire to have more. The serving dish on the table is an unspoken suggestion to eat more, which your unconscious mind picks up on and manufactures desire. But, remove the suggestion, and "poof!" The desire diminishes. That is what we are after, to control what we have been unable to control by sheer will.

What kind of suggestions are you presented with each day? Are there donuts next to the coffee machine? Chocolates at the nurse's station? It suggests that eating those things casually is normal and expected. Untrue! Ask anyone who works to control their weight. Those trappings are the hallmark of a sick, indulgent, obese life. It is up to you to meet those suggestions with your own self-talk, saying, "No way am I buying into the promotion of obesity and all the illness that goes with it. That is a sick way of life, and we need to quit it."

REFRAMING

Think back and remember my point about CBT (Cognitive Behavior Therapy) being based on the idea that the way we feel is not a result of events, but the way we think about the events. While it is hard to get control of our feelings (including feeling like eating), it is possible to control the way we think, which will, in turn, affect the way we feel.

Reframing is the practice of changing the meaning of something, looking at it in a new way, in a new frame, so that the meaning of the thing changes.

The flat tire is a good example. If you look at it as a disaster, proof that the world and the universe is out to get you, you'll feel miserable. If you look at it as an inconvenience, and a good thing that it happened where it did rather than someplace far worse, you won't feel so bad— especially when you remind yourself that you are not in a war zone, which many others deal with on a daily basis. It's not the event so much as the way you think about it that will influence the way you feel.

One of the really useful applications of this technique is related to the issue of hunger. When you undereat, you will feel hungry. It's not a terrible thing, but it will happen and will then cause something else to happen. Usually, when we feel hungry, we think "It's time to eat," a powerful suggestion. We might say, "I'm starving. I've got to eat," or "I should eat. The dietitian told me to listen to my body, so, it's OK to eat."

Instead, when you feel that twinge of hunger, think "Oh… That means I've burned up all the calories from my last meal, and now I'm burning fat! Burn, baby, burn! The only way I'm going to get what I want is to burn the fat off my body, and if I eat something, I'll stop it. I'm finally getting the job done. Hunger means I'm burning the fat. Keep burning!"

It's silly to be afraid of being hungry, as if it's going to kill you, thinking that one has to stop that feeling. If you have that attitude, you'll be hypnotizing yourself to eat and be unable to control what happens.

The way we think of the scale is another example of reframing, changing the way we think about something, what it means to us. The scale doesn't lie? Bull! The scale *doesn't* give us honest feedback on a day-to-day or week-to-week basis. Your calorie log is the only way to tell how you did today. "The scale lies! I know I only ate one thousand calories today, and I burn 1,800! I burned off a stick of butter today, and I'll burn another off tomorrow!"

When you've been imperfect and eaten something you hadn't planned on, don't label it a failure, where you've "blown it" or "broken the spell." It's just some calories over what you had planned on. So, you didn't hit a home run today? Big deal. You can still have a pretty good win. My most successful clients have days that don't go well. I do, too. But it's part of the twenty-three years of success I've had. Frame your imperfections in a new way. They are not proof of your hopelessness. They are proof of your humanity, simply a mistake, the same kind that all successful people have made.

Reframing will give you a lot of opportunities to practice therapeutic self-talk.

Examine how you look at things and what you've been saying to yourself about them. With any events or conditions that are troublesome in your life, see if there is a different way you can look at them, or frame them, so they are cast in a different light. Even something as traumatic as the death of a loved one can take on a more healing character when it is seen as a release from the world of suffering, a natural progression through the existence that we all face, rather than a cruel insult.

EXAMINING AND CHANGING BELIEF SYSTEMS

Our system of beliefs about ourselves and our world, and the way things are, is probably the most powerful psychogenic phenomena that exist.

Albert Ellis, a psychologist who played a huge part in the development of cognitive behavior therapy, pointed out that a lot of the thinking we have that causes emotional and psychological problems isn't even true or rational. He led his clients to stop their irrational thinking to eliminate a lot of the bad feelings they have.

For instance, it's common for people to say things like "I never get anything right," or "No matter what I do, I gain weight." Then, we immediately feel like failures, hopeless, worthless, and angry. We actually get ourselves to believe that it's true.

Ellis pointed out that these things aren't even true. We were lying to ourselves. No one "*never* gets anything right." Did you put the shoes on the wrong feet? Did you drive on the wrong side of the road? There are probably *millions* of things you got right before you made a mistake, but then, when you made one mistake, you said, "I always screw up," and felt like a total failure.

You can't lose weight? Wrong. If you figure out how to eat fewer calories habitually, you'll lose weight, and if you don't stop, you'll starve to death. The truth is, you haven't done that yet. Just because it hasn't happened yet does not mean that it will not, unless you make it so. It is not true or rational to say things like "No matter what I do, I gain weight," because when you eat fewer calories than you burn, you'll lose weight. I guarantee it. Stop saying things to yourself that are not true or rational. They will make you feel awful, and the awful feeling is as real as anything you have experienced in life, as you well know.

Start saying, "Its hard work to succeed, but other former food addicts have figured it out, and when I do, too, I'll succeed, just like them." That would be true, and you'd feel better, too. Start saying, "Oops. I made a mistake. Just like every other human being on the planet, I am not perfect yet. I'll learn, and I'll get better." That would be true, and you'll feel better, too.

Ellis proved to people that they could alter the reality of their emotional life by paying attention to what they thought and said, what they believed, and eliminating what was nonsense.

If you say or think, "I have to go to work," if that's what you believe, you end up feeling oppressed and powerless. The truth is you don't "have to." No one is holding a gun to your head. You can choose to stay home, if you are willing to accept the results. The truth is, it is your choice whether to go to work today, whether to stay in that job, that marriage, etc. etc. etc. When you stop pretending you have no choice and get honest that you have the power to make the choices in what to do and what not to do, you feel more powerful, more able to fashion a life more fair and satisfying, if you are willing to do the work.

Ellis and others, like David Burns, developed detailed plans with which we can look at the ways we think and believe, to see what is irrational and dysfunctional. They wrote books to show us how to identify the thinking habits we have that make us feel bad and change them. As I said before, I think CBT is the most significant contribution to psychotherapy since the term was coined.

THE CHALLENGE

From our earliest days, we develop the way we think, the way we look at the world, and what we believe, and until we are challenged to question it, we tend to believe that we have a handle on the truth. We tend to think that the way we think, habitually, is the only way, the only "take" on reality. It is not. Many of the thinking habits that you may have developed may completely misrepresent the life you are able to experience. Your early teachers may not have had a good handle on things themselves, so what you learned from them will include their mistakes. It is time to leave them and find your own way.

I pointed out earlier that advertisers and propagandists count on the fact that if you say something enough times, it will begin to feel true. Many of the things you may believe, that feel true, are not. You have simply thought them over and over again, habitually, and your mind has accepted them as if you were hypnotized.

I had been overweight my whole life, since I was seven, and whenever I tried to diet, I failed. No matter what I did, I kept gaining weight. It didn't seem that I ate more than others. We all liked to eat! My father's side of the family was all "big people," and it seemed that I "took after them." My parents, the authorities, confirmed these "facts."

I said things like "No matter what, I keep gaining weight." "I was born to be fat." "I'll never get this weight off." I said these things over and over again.

When I was told that I could lose weight, like anyone else, something inside me completely rejected this. It conflicted with what I "knew" was true. I would have sworn on a stack of bibles that it was my "nature" to be fat and that I would gain weight on the same diet that others would succeed with.

My belief systems were firmly set. I trusted them and knew them to be true like I trusted that I knew my own name. But they were phony as a three dollar bill. I had hypnotized myself into beliefs that were false, and those belief systems created the reality that I was living with.

Our beliefs, what we have come to believe is true, become the things that we imagine and expect, unconsciously, twenty-four/seven. If they are based on a lie, on something irrational and unhealthy, our wonderful computer-like mind/body will be working twenty-four/seven to create something unhealthy.

The truth is, God or nature, however you frame it, made none of us to be fat. Look around at the other creatures: the deer, the squirrels, the big cats. None of them are obese. Your body was designed to be fit. Your skeleton and organ systems are designed to support only so much girth, and no more. Our being fat is a mistake. It is not your nature. It is a lie to believe it, even if it feels true now.

What do you believe about what is possible, about what you deserve in life, about how the world and reality works? If what you have believed is wrong, and it is less than what is possible, it would be a shame, because you will be limited to experiencing only what you believe. What if the real higher truth is that all things are possible, and that you are due a life of blessings and health and happiness, a kind of heaven on earth? One thing for certain, it would only start to feel true after you've heard it more than the old stuff.

To change the unhealthy, irrational thinking habits and erroneous belief systems, it will take a lot of work. You start by deciding to believe in a higher truth. Look around. Listen for it. But then, when you find it, you must brainwash yourself with it, think it over and over again; say it, read it, hear it, again and again, until it feels true, until *the* truth becomes *your* truth. It will be work, but it will be worth it.

CHAPTER 13

The Prerequisites

With my method, the first session with a client costs them nothing. It's a no-charge consultation. They get to find out a bit about the approach, and we learn a bit about them.

We want to make sure they have no misunderstandings about what they are engaging in and what they will need to contribute in order to expect a good outcome.

Sometimes, people are under the impression that a good weight loss program should be easy. Some think that they are hiring someone to solve a problem for them, like a repairman. Then, they think, it is the repairman's responsibility to fix the problem. They think that somehow, because they are paying, we will make them successful without they, themselves, needing to do much. After all, psychotherapists don't come cheap. We don't charge as much as doctors or lawyers charge, but still, it's nothing to sneeze at. I had one prospective client say "For that amount, I shouldn't have to do *any*thing," as if paying enough should get him whatever he wanted, and by paying, he should be able to make up the rules of how we'd do things.

What you get with The Anderson Method is not something that you can get by paying money. You must give something much more significant. It's like learning to swim, or ride a bike, or use a computer; no one else can do it for you. Someone else can help and teach, but you must do the work, and unless you make certain contributions to the effort, you'll never see the result.

So, we make it clear that there are some prerequisites that must be met, some contributions that you must make, and some terms that you must irrevocably agree to in order to get what you've come for. After we've talked a bit, and we determine that you are a promising candidate, we ask if you are able to make these contributions. If you can't, we don't go any further. If you can, we begin the work.

So, here is what you must agree to before you can start to succeed:

SOLVING THIS PROBLEM IS THE PRIORITY.

Nothing can come before your health and weight control. It must be *the* most important thing. Nothing can get in the way of what you must do to succeed at this. Not the job. Not the family. Not church. Not friends. Nothing. It's got to be number one, numero uno.

Some people have been critical of this, saying that it's out of balance and sick. I understand what they are concerned about. I agree that our lives need to be properly centered and balanced, and we will address that issue before you finish the book. But you will not be able to solve this problem, nor do what the method will require of you, by putting in a half measure. In the first months especially, you will need to put in one hundred percent, and whenever there is a conflict between what needs to be done to work the program and something or someone else, you need to choose your health and the work, and the other thing must take a back seat to it.

Some clients have thought that they will do what's required "unless something at work comes up," or unless some family event interferes, or unless a church issue or a relationship issue makes it difficult. Surely, they think, I didn't mean that weight control and the work would come before *those* things, did I?

Yes. That's exactly what I meant. Your health and weight control, and the work in the program to attain it, must come before any and all of those things.

Losing the weight and solving your weight problem must be your top priority. Your health and well-being must be the most important things in your life. Everything else can be considered and attended to after, as long you can do what needs to be done to maintain your health first, and not before.

HONESTY

Earlier, I spoke of how we can lie to ourselves, and how we can unknowingly screw ourselves up by having irrational and erroneous beliefs. It is amazing how common it is to mess up our "computer" with bad data. There is an old axiom in computer circles, "garbage in, garbage out." Nowhere is this more evident than in our own mind and our battle with obesity.

The first line of defense for all addicts is denial, and overweight people and dieters are masters of denial. What do you say when you are asked what your weight is? I'll ask you right now, and I'll bet your answer is way off if you go and get on a scale. And there's no one else here you're even trying to fool!

Have you ever said things like "I don't eat that much," or "No matter what I do, I don't lose weight?" Saying these things is not being honest. The truth is, you eat more than you need to maintain a healthy weight. If you were to eat less than you burn, I *guarantee* that you would begin to burn your body fat and lose weight. When you said those things, you were not being honest.

When someone asks what you eat, like the doctor or dietician, do you tell them about an ideal day, or do you tell them about your normal overeating days? *Don't lie now!* You've probably looked them right in the eye, and told them about your "good" days, not the "bad" ones.

When you have dieted, have you ever measured out just a little more, and then pretended you followed the diet? We even lie to ourselves!

Now, don't feel too guilty. It's normal. How do you think I know about all this stuff? I'm better now because I changed, but before I got better, I did this stuff, just like all my clients.

The point is, we've got to quit it to be able to solve this problem.

In order to succeed, we need to develop a scrupulous regard for the truth. We need to catch ourselves saying those dishonest little things we say all the time and stop it. We need to be honest with ourselves, and our helpers. Otherwise, we won't get very far.

In order to solve this problem we need to become scrupulously honest.

It has less to do with moral purity than with sanity. We need to stop playing fast and loose with the truth because when we are careless with it, we lose track of it ourselves. We remember the stories we made up rather than what really happened. We believe in the lie, and we don't even know we've lost touch with reality. We store bad data in our subconscious computer, and then that wonderful twenty-four/seven autopilot becomes useless to us. Even if we got it to attempt to take us to our dreams, it's got the wrong info on how to get there, if we haven't been careful with the truth.

Unless we get honest with ourselves and others, it's a lost cause, hopeless. Being honest is an absolute prerequisite. And that includes meaning what you say.

This is an absolute requirement: No bull****.

MATURE RESPONSIBILITY

This makes everyone shudder. It's a frightening prospect, growing up, getting mature.

I'm not suggesting, however, that you need to be perfect and never fail to carry out everything you attempt.

I'm talking about owning what you do.

I've had business guys tell me they had to drink to do business. "It was an important client and an important lunch meeting. I really had no choice." I imagine they had guns and held him down while they forced the martinis and lasagna on him.

I've had people say that it was just not possible to eat a little and maintain any friendships or social life. "I can't stop having lunch with my friends," as if their friends were forcing them to eat a lot.

We've got to stop pretending that others or the circumstances are forcing us, that *they* are responsible. We need to be honest and say "Nobody made me. I'm the one who did it."

We need to grow up and take responsibility for our actions, instead of blaming someone or something else.

There may be circumstances that make things difficult, but blaming them won't help. If we want something, *we* are the one who must make it happen. No one else can take the job of being the cause of what we want. We need to accept that job.

Mature responsibility means taking an ownership role in your life. Owning what you do. Owning what you did. Owning the job before you.

WILLINGNESS TO MAKE EFFORT, TO WORK.

When a client signs up, we make these terms clear, and we even have a written agreement they read and sign, so there are no misunderstandings.

There is work to be done. There is homework. There is reading. We explain that there is nothing beyond their capability, but the homework must be done, and there is no one checking on them, so they need to be honest about it.

It may have been years since they studied, or maybe they never really studied, getting through school on the least amount of work possible. That won't work with this project. They will need to really read, like reading a textbook— no getting by by coasting. Being "smart" may be a hindrance. It's effort that will pay off, not understanding by itself, or intellectualism.

One client, a teacher, said that she hadn't had to pay so much attention to anything since grad school, talking as if grad school was more important and deserved real effort, where this shouldn't. I said that she had misunderstood. I told her that to win her weight control dream, it had to be *more* important than grad school, and she had to give it *more* attention, not less. You could see it sink in, and she did well.

Clients may not understand the reasons for the assignments or agree that what we ask of them makes sense, but we will not work with someone who wants to pick and choose what to do. Clients will not get the results of technique that they do not use. We don't explain why they are doing what we tell them, not at first anyway. We just give them assignments, and those who do them come back with surprising results.

Sometimes the homework takes up to an hour a day, so if your schedule is full, something else will have to go to make time for the work.

Clients who have become accustomed to buying services to fit their convenience are sometimes thrown by this. They want a way that won't take much time, or that won't be a bother, as if they think they can hire someone to do it for them.

This is one of those areas of life where you can't hire someone to do the work for you. You can only succeed by your own efforts. Being very rich or "smart" won't help. You will only get what you want if you are willing to do the work.

FOLLOWING

Frankly, some of the technique seems silly, or nonsensical, or unlikely to do any good, in the client's opinion. We don't explain the theories behind the technique, not at first, anyway. We don't try to persuade people to do the work, either. We just make it clear what they need to do for homework, all of which anyone with a seventh grade education can do, and we expect them to do it.

Clients often have had a habit of, when given instructions at school or work, choosing which ones they will follow, almost with the attitude that "no one really does all this stuff. You only do the minimum to get by." That won't work with this. They will not get the result they are looking for if they selectively follow.

We explain that they will get a happy result if they can assume the attitude of a real student, an eager apprentice, and follow everything, no matter how foolish or useless it may seem. While we need to be mature, if we can retain the child's ability to play follow-the-leader or Simon Says, we will get a great payoff. Trying to get by on the cheap will cause problems you don't need to have.

One of the main prerequisites is the agreement to suspend the ego and just follow. It can work miracles.

CAN *YOU* MAKE THESE CONTRIBUTIONS?

Yes, of course you can.

You may not want to yet, but you can. The difference between someone who can't give of these things and someone who can can be measured in milliseconds. It's a decision.

CHAPTER 14

What Do You Really *Need?*

The light from the refrigerator was dimly illuminating the room, and there I was, with one hand on the door, peering in, trying to figure out what it was that I needed.

It was just one of my overeating habits, but it was the one that most truly demonstrated the strange and powerful drive I knew as *craving*. Sometimes I didn't even know what it was I was craving. I just knew that I *needed* something, and I was looking for it. At times, I would crave specific things. At other times, I just craved, but I didn't know what.

I was sure I'd find it in the fridge, or in the cupboards. If I didn't find it on the first pass, I'd go back and look again, to see if I could spot it this time. I would always find *some*thing, and it felt like it was what I needed, but then, after a while, I'd be back there again, surveying the shelves.

"I just *need* something," I'd say, and others would say, "You just ate an hour ago. You *can't* be hungry," but I was.

I knew I needed something. The craving wouldn't quiet until I ate.

NEEDS AND CRAVING

Craving is a natural phenomenon. It is desire on the "high" setting. It can be triggered by the absence of something we've become addicted to, an acquired need, or it can be triggered by the absence of a natural need, like food or water. If we go without a need met, we will feel desire, then craving, and we will have no peace until we satisfy it.

WHAT DO YOU REALLY NEED?

Psychologists have theorized that our motivation, the power to make us move and act, our *drive*, can be explained as *needs reduction,* the drive to reduce or eliminate our sense of need.

It's as if we are born incomplete. We're missing something. For us to survive and be fully functioning human beings, we must obtain whatever it is that's missing, what we need. We will feel an emptiness, a craving, until we've gotten it.

The moment we are born, we begin our lifelong quest to satisfy need, our lifelong experience of desire and craving. We start with the food that satisfies our hunger pangs, but food, of course, is not our only need. We will be driven to satisfy all of our needs until we are complete, and we will not stop until they are met. Need and craving will be a constant companion until it is done.

There are those who say they need nothing, and when all our needs are met, it is true. We are complete. We need nothing. But that wasn't me.

I knew I needed something, and I thought it would be in the fridge.

EMOTIONAL EATING AND COMFORT FOOD?

It has become cliché.

I found it irritating, even as a kid, when dieticians thought they were revealing some great discovery in pointing out that we eat for reasons other than physical hunger. They said we should ask ourselves if we were eating because we were hungry or for some emotional reason.

They thought that if we knew we were eating to comfort hurt feelings, or because we were lonely or depressed, then voila, the problem was solved, as if then, with this insight, we wouldn't need to eat. Wrong. I still craved the food, and the food still worked to make me feel better.

We use food to satisfy a whole bunch of needs it was never meant to satisfy. One of the main problems with this is that it seems to work! It feels better. It feels like the need is being satisfied.

In some cases, the food actually *does* satisfy the emotional need.

Imagine we have been conditioned, like Pavlov's dog, to experience being comforted when we eat cookies and milk. Imagine that over and over, many times, we ate cookies and milk, and at the same time, we basked in our family's comforting love. Now, just like the dog that salivates when he hears the bell, our brain actually "feels the love" when we eat the cookies. The brain plays the "feeling loved" program, just like it plays the "salivate" program. It actually works!

Knowing that we are eating for reasons that have nothing to do with physical hunger or need does very little in solving the problem, even when we know what the real need is.

Certainly, knowing what we need helps a great deal. Then, we can work to have the real need satisfied with the real stuff. We can take steps, for example, to engage in relationships where we experience love, giving, and receiving. If we don't, and instead we just go after the cookies when we feel that need, not only will we get fat, but we will prevent ourselves from truly satisfying our real need for loving relationships.

Being conscious of what we really need as human beings can help us move toward real wholeness, to become more complete human beings. This possibility gives us even more reasons to address our attachments and addictions.

One of the theories regarding attachments and addictions is that they are substitutes for what we truly need, like love, or comforting, and that to break the power of an addiction, we need to seek real satisfaction of the need. Then the power of the addiction weakens. If we only indulge in the addiction without attempting to fulfill what it is pretending to satisfy, we will be indulging in something that will never fulfill us. We will be slaves to craving and consuming something without end, never satisfied—but stuck with the results of the addiction. Whether the addiction is food, drugs, alcohol, sex, gambling, money, power, work, the internet, or any number of other unhealthy addictions, we will be addicted and sick with it, still feeling empty, no closer to getting what we really need. Addiction is an obstacle that we need to break through in order to be truly satisfied.

Making sure we get our real needs met holds the promise of real fulfillment, a solution to the craving and emptiness, and freedom from the power of the addiction.

Does getting our real need satisfied, for example, for love or comforting, make it so we don't care for cookies and milk anymore?

No. I can't say that all my old "friends," like cookies and cake and ice cream, or cashews and margaritas, have lost their appeal, but they have lost power. By making sure that I'm attending to my real needs, and working to make sure they are satisfied with the real stuff, I have gained a position where those old buddies are no longer *the* power in my life. They still may call, but I am no longer powerless to deal with it.

Making sure we attend to our real needs not only holds the promise of breaking the hold of the addiction, but it also holds out the promise of real fulfillment, an end to the emptiness.

Clients who have succeeded in controlling their weight often say they have gotten so much *more* from learning my method.

They say that their lives are richer, not just because they have solved their weight problem, but that their lives have become much fuller in other ways.

To solve your weight problem, you must become familiar with your real needs as a human being, not just what it *feels* like you crave, but what you *really* need to be fully human, with all your needs met. Only when you attend to that will you break the power of your unhealthy attachments and addictions.

It's not OK to keep getting something to eat when it feels like something is missing. We need to start getting the real stuff.

Examine with me some of the ideas about what those needs are, what some others think, and then you can decide what you'll do about it.

SCIENCE OR NONSCIENCE?

Years ago, in my first clinical psychology courses that addressed the subjects of addiction and alcoholism, I was surprised to find that there was almost no mention of Alcoholics Anonymous. The only mention of AA seemed to minimize any role it might have in addressing these disorders. AA was pretty much dismissed as a support group. The professors talked about different effective psychotherapies to address those problems, but AA was dismissed as unprofessional and without merit.

I wasn't really aware of much about AA, other than hearing about it occasionally in the community. Hearing what these teachers said, I assumed that AA actually wasn't much of a help to anyone. After all, I thought, if it was really of any value, the teachers who were teaching prospective therapists would give us an accurate picture of what helped people.

Later, when I started working in the clinical settings that actually provided treatment to addicts and alcoholics, I learned that almost all effective treatment was centered on AA and its principles. It seemed that every legitimate treatment center and clinical team hooked people up with AA and led them to the plan of recovery they called the "Twelve Steps."

Why was AA downplayed by the academics when it was universally accepted as the only game in town by the clinical community that worked with these disorders?

At first, I thought it was because AA was not a part of the academic community. It was not run by people with the letters after their names, and it did not involve paying credentialed people for services.

But that was not the main reason. It turns out that AA is a *spiritual* plan of recovery. It was a kind of religion. The Twelve Steps they talked about included turning your life and will over to a Higher Power, God; it included things like prayer and forgiveness.

Wow.

No wonder my New England university-based science professors steered clear of AA. There was no way they could introduce the idea of a religious conversion as psychotherapy, and at the same time propose that their psychology and psychotherapy was "science."

Religious people think that our real need is for God and right relationship with God, and some think that all addictions are a substitute for that, false Gods. They think that until we get right with God and fill that spiritual need, we will not be able to be free of those addictions. If we put God first, all our other needs will be met. AA was closer to those religious ideas than it was to psychotherapy.

University-based scholars have been struggling for years to make the study of the mind "scientific." They want "psychology" to be as scientific, in terms of reliability and method, as the hard sciences, like chemistry and physics. They want to be on par with other scientists, with their rules of evidence, where you can use scales and microscopes to prove things. I don't think that will ever happen. You just can't put the psyche, the mind or soul, under a microscope.

So, the subject ends up being a matter of faith, where you must decide what to believe. That being said, here's what the psychologists (the majority) think:

HIERARCHY OF NEEDS

The names are legendary in the field of psychology: Freud, Jung, Adler, Fromm, Allport, Rogers, Maslow, Frankl. All observed our motives and strivings, our needs and state of need; and they described or implied a needless state, where our sense of need is satisfied. Presumably, this would be a state without craving. Taken as a whole, they seem to propose that we make our way through a "hierarchy" of needs, where, as we experience a need and satisfy it, we then become aware of a new, higher need. When we satisfy that higher need, we then become aware of an even higher need. As we make our way through this hierarchy, we are not conscious or aware of the higher needs until the lower ones are satisfied.

For instance, the lower needs are the physical survival needs: for food, water, shelter, freedom from pain, etc. Social needs, such as the need for companionship, and the need to be liked or loved by others, would be thought of as higher needs.

If we are starving or dying of thirst, the higher social needs don't get any attention. We want food and water, and if others get in the way, watch out. We don't want company, and we don't care if we are liked. We want the food and water, and if we need to clobber someone to get it, so be it.

If our lower needs are met, if we have all the food we need, and our material and physical needs are met, and our future is secure, we start to experience a need for something else. We crave the company of others; we want to be liked; we may crave their approval and acceptance.

When we were starving, we didn't give a hoot about companionship or being accepted. We didn't have that need, and we weren't even aware that it might become a need. We may have scoffed at the idea. But, as the lower needs were satisfied, the higher needs began to emerge and assert their power. We'd satisfy the lower needs, and with that done, we begin to feel a new desire for something else; and when that becomes fulfilled with friendships and a sense of acceptance and belonging, then *another* higher set of needs begins to emerge. And so on.

The idea is that we would progress, hopefully, through this hierarchy to a place where we are totally satisfied, with all our needs met, complete and without unfulfilled need. Or we might not. If we get stuck at a low level, and don't get that lower need fulfilled, we don't progress. Starving people are not going to be concerned with much else until they get that problem solved. Hopefully, when we get a lower need satisfied, we become aware of the higher need instead of getting stuck on the lower ones, or, God forbid, create more, as we do with drug addictions.

What are these lower and higher needs that we should be aware of?

If we want any chance at all of getting to the peak of the hierarchy, it will help to know what they are.

LOWER NEEDS

I always thought of the basic animal needs we all have when they talked of lower needs. These are the survival needs, the physical needs, like the need for food, water, shelter, and warmth if it's cold. The word "lower" made me think of them as primal, primitive, base— lower and crude— needs of the body, as opposed to higher and loftier needs of the mind or soul, the part of us that is not simply body.

The deprivation of our survival needs can trigger awesome craving and truly bestial behavior. Think of the behavior of drowning people, clawing at their rescuers, or the people fighting over the water given out in the wake of disasters. The need for a breath of air, water, and food becomes our only need when we are denied them, and nothing else counts. There are no other needs until they are met.

Our physical needs include sex, absolutely necessary for the survival of species, and freedom from pain. Pain, stress, and illness, whether it is from an injury, withdrawal of an addictive drug, or another type of trauma, can disable us, render us incapable of seeing to our other survival needs. Pain, like starvation, can become the overriding motivator in a person's life, so that nothing else exists for them except securing relief, and they will do whatever it takes to obtain it.

Some would like to deny that sex is a need, out of some misguided view of reality, but common sense tell us that for a culture to exist over time, sex is required just as much as food. Observation of real people throughout history has led many casual observers, as well as scientists, to conclude that the sex drive is our most powerful drive. Freud thought that sexual drive was the central experience of our life force, expressing itself as a need for pleasure, and if it was not expressed sexually, it would somehow seek other expression. (Is the pleasure of eating comparable?)

Is pleasure a need? You bet.

Go without pleasure too long, and you'll get sick. You'll get depressed, and your brain chemistry will change. You may need medication to right it, and to get better, you'll need to make sure you start getting some pleasure in your life— and in our case, it needs to be something without calories.

Chances are, you've satisfied your lower needs. Otherwise you wouldn't be reading this.

But your need for food is the only need you should be using food for, and at this moment, it may not be.

If you're going to change how you eat, and you've been using food to satisfy one of your other needs, change is not going to happen without attending to that need. That's why it's called a "need." Something in you will start clawing and fighting, like the drowning man.

If eating is the only pleasure you've been getting, you are going to need to figure out what else to do.

Sex and exercise (which really surprised me) seem to be the main things that people depend on for pleasure when they are trying to limit using food. There are others that work, though not so visceral.

Fortunately, we don't have to altogether give up food or enjoying it. In fact, most clients enjoy their eating more than ever; but we will need other pleasures to lessen our dependence on eating.

Are you depressed? Are you treating it? In many cases, people who are depressed and resisting the use of antidepressant medications are self-medicating with food, though it does a poor job. Again, if you've been using food for this, and you want to change, you'll need to attend to your brain's call for some adjustment of the neurotransmitters.

Is eating your stress management technique? It can be a beauty. Works like a charm. I know people who can de-stress in the wink of an eye, like going into a trance, when they sit down with a snack. They have relaxed and snacked at the same time, so many times, that relaxing is a conditioned response to eating, like the bladder relaxing to the sound of running water. If this is what you've done, you'll need to develop a new stress reduction technique if you want to be able to change the way you use food. If you try to do without a daily relaxation session that you need as much as a junkie needs a fix, you'll fail. You don't need to snack every day, but you do need to de-stress every day.

If you're ill or in pain, you may have been using food as a pain killer or comfort, and that is a real Catch Twenty-two. You use eating to feel better, and in many cases, it is the very thing that causes the illness and pain. I have seen miracles when people have decided to lose weight as a part of their plan to deal with their illness and pain. They may have gone years neglecting their health, with no interest in changing their weight. When they've had enough of feeling sick, and they commit themselves to beating the illness and pain, I've seen a lot of success, even though eating has been the main way they responded to it. They lock arms with their doctors, take the medications precisely, and focus on reducing the excess body weight that has been complicating everything. They love seeing their doctor and getting all the test results as they improve. Getting better and taking medications correctly is a far better way to respond to illness and pain than overeating.

As I said, if you are reading this book, your lower needs have been met. No one who is struggling to survive can give their attention to anything but getting the day's meal, having a roof over their head, staying warm, and fighting to survive. If those things are satisfied, the next level emerges.

SAFETY AND SECURITY NEEDS

When we've satisfied our most basic survival needs, we start thinking about how we will continue to satisfy them, how to guarantee their continuance. We become concerned with feeling secure and safe, the needs that move into our awareness when we've done what we need to do to survive.

For primitive cultures, safety and security might have come from living in a strong tribe, in a defendable fort, in a land with abundant game and edible vegetation.

Today, people may feel secure with money in the bank, or a lucrative profession, in a community with law and order and a strong defense. For some, having health insurance gives them a sense of security, and for others, it's having a gun handy.

However you satisfy it, you have a need to feel that things will be OK. You'll be motivated to do something to rid yourself of the fear or anxiety that they won't be. You'll need to relax, even if it's only for the night, and feel reasonably sure that things will be OK.

Some have the attitude that they can handle whatever comes along— they fear nothing and are ready for anything. Others depend on these people, and it is their faith in them that makes them feel secure. For some, it's their faith in a loving God and their belief that everything will be OK in the end, regardless of what life hands them.

However you satisfy it, you have a need to do something that makes you feel OK when your sense of security and safety is threatened.

Does food play any part here?

It certainly did when we emerged from the womb, rudely thrust from our serene existence into a cold, noisy, chaotic, and frightening nightmare. We were put to the breast, and calmed, and began life learning that our survival and safety was in the arms of a God called "mother," who was, coincidently, also our food, one and the same.

As we grew, for many of us, our home and family was our security. And our experience of family was felt most deeply at our meals, whether they were ordinary breakfasts and dinners, or our most important holidays.

From day one, when we felt our only security while we ate, through our childhood years and beyond, we have been conditioned, like Pavlov's dog, to feel secure and safe each time we ate. With each meal, we were made to feel "*comfort*able," thousands and thousands of times. It would be a miracle if eating *didn't* make you feel secure and safe.

If you want to make sure your "needing something to eat" is not an answer to your need for a sense of safety and security, you will need to look at this issue of security and what you depend on to feel safe and secure. While food might work for a moment, it really doesn't do the job, and there's that caloric side effect!

Do you feel secure? If so, why? In this world of uncertainty and threat, what satisfies your need for some peace and security? If you don't feel secure, what will you do to satisfy it? What will you turn to?

SOCIAL NEEDS

I'm not the only one who has referred to a certain food as an old friend or buddy. In fact, I think most of my clients have had the same experience. Oreos and milk, or donuts and coffee, or potato chips and coke, have seemed like a friend that they could depend on, always there if they were needed.

When overeaters, and smokers, too, try to quit their habit, they often report that they feel like they have lost a friend. When the world was cold and heartless, and they withdrew from the world to their lair, their "old friend" was always there to greet them. Breaking away, for many, was a loss that they could not tolerate.

In those cases, it's almost as if the food filled, or pretended to fill, one of the social needs we have, the set of needs that emerges once our security and safety needs are answered in some way.

These are the needs that have to do with friendship, companionship, family, and our relationship to our greater family down the road and around the globe. It is the need for love, the need to be accepted and loved by others. It is the need to feel that you belong to something greater than yourself, that you are a part of something, something big, something that is *for* you, that has a special place for you.

Our desire and satisfaction of this need is what drives us to seek out friends, to please them, to avoid being rejected and criticized by others, to have companions and join groups and societies. While affection is physical, it is also a bonding and expression of mutual acceptance with another. Friends, lovers, family, church, clubs, neighborhoods— these all answer our social needs; and sometimes, our old buddies, like cookies and milk, fill that spot.

How are you satisfying your social needs? It's hard enough to break the overeating habits, but if your "old friends," like my Oreos and milk, are the only ones you can count on at the end of the day, it will be impossible to break the addiction. Something in you will drive you, and your social needs *will* be answered.

EGO NEEDS

When we need approval from others, is it really a social need, or is it something else? Some say that we need others to say that we are OK because then, and only then, we are able to believe it ourselves. While we need to feel accepted by others, we also have a need to feel OK about ourselves. This is one of the "ego" needs, the need to have a sense of who and what we are and to feel good about it.

We have a need for identity, to have an idea of who we are, a self-concept and a self-image— and we have a need to like it, to have self-esteem. It is a need to like ourselves, to *love* ourselves.

This can be a real problem for a guy or gal who thinks "I'm a slob, a miserable failure. I hate myself."

You may think that you know yourself, that what you are has already been formed, but look at how wrong you've been about other things. You may be wrong about that, too.

The wisest among us have proposed that our main problem is that we've forgotten who we are, that we've lost touch with our real "self," and that we've believed in a delusion, a mistaken belief about our self. They think that many of us, after we were born, were influenced by misguided teachers, perhaps flawed parents, or maybe the TV, a culture that we were born into and believed in, but a culture that was absolutely wrong-headed about things.

This will be something that you'll have to look at and decide about. What do you really believe? Who and what are you?

Are you your body, or are you the person who has the body, the mind and soul that lives in one?

Are you a collection of habits? Or are you the person who *has* the habits?

Are you a child, a parent, a boss, a worker, a success, a failure, a character in the play that is your life? Are you the role in this play, or are you the actor, the person who has been playing this role?

Consider the proposition that we are controlled by that which we identify with, and we are able to control that which we have identified is *not* us. This would have us believe that if we think we are simply a bunch of habits, then the habits control things; but if we believe that we are a person who *has* the habits, then *we* can be in control, able to add and delete the ones we want to change, able to change roles. If we were to delete our habits, and we believed that we are nothing but a collection of habits, then where are we? Gone? Dead?

No, we can't change what we really are. But, we can change the circumstances that we find ourselves in. So, we'd better get it right when we decide what we are, what the "self" really is. It is not your body, fat or thin. It is not your habits, good or bad. It is not the role you play, whether it is bad child or good child, bad parent or good parent. It is not boss, servant, butcher, baker, or candlestick maker.

You are the actor playing the role, not the role itself. You are the creator of the part you have played, and you need to be in touch with that nature of creation, the love that it has for the created. Those are your ego needs.

You have a need for a self-concept, a self-image, and a need to "know thyself"— and everyone reading this will recognize the inherent truth in this: You are the soul or spirit that inhabits your body, the being and energy that generates it and lives in it.

You are the person who has the habits, good or bad, who has the body, healthy or unhealthy. And you can change those things, because they are not the real you.

You are a human being with a mind and spirit of a creative nature, endowed with an energy and will that delights in pleasure and love, capable of all sorts of miraculous things, but a human being nonetheless, who can sometimes be lost and confused.

You are challenged to find the truth about yourself and be open to possibilities that fly in the face of what you've been taught to believe. You have been raised by a culture that once told its children that the earth is flat and that the sun revolves around it. What you have come to believe about yourself may be just as false, whether it is that you are fat, average, a "consumer," "just like your mother/father," or any number of false things. It's not true that the earth is flat, that you can't teach an old dog new tricks, or that "you'll never amount to anything," as one of our greatest leaders, Lincoln, was told as a child.

You are the thing that says "I am _____," and you are to develop it, and completely accept it, let it be as great as it can be, whatever that is, and treat it with absolute love and respect. Those are your ego needs.

It's said that our needs for recognition, professional success, social position, and self-esteem are ego needs, and that is true. But there is more to it. Read on.

SELF-ACTUALIZATION NEEDS

This appears to be an oxymoron. When the psychologists describe a "self-actualizing" person, they talk about someone who is no longer working to satisfy needs, but someone who is instead, happily "being," being genuine, letting a "Real Self" emerge and unfold.

They talk about transcending the ego, and living not just for themselves, but for a higher purpose, as a part of something greater— loving the self, but also giving the self.

They talk about "coming to terms" with the Cosmos, accepting one's place in it, and satisfying a need for meaning in life, something important. They talk about being a part of something greater than one's self and yielding to it.

Sounds kind of like what the spiritual people were talking about.

Could food or other addictions pretend to satisfy this, too?

One of the most insidious features of an addiction is the way it can worm its way into life, so that it becomes the most important thing, where it is the last thing that would go. Addicts' lives can revolve around getting and using, and anything that threatens the habit crumbles almost as soon as it appears.

When I learned that in order to avoid being overweight, I would have to give up, forever, the freedom to eat whatever I wanted when I got home, I panicked. When I dieted, I always held onto the belief that eventually the weight loss would end, and I could return to unconscious eating-at-will. Having learned the truth about caloric balance and the eating habits I had developed, I learned that was not an option.

When I realized I would have to live without my freedom to eat whatever I wanted when I got home, I thought "If I have to live without that, what's the point?" Many of my clients have had this feeling. Had eating become our purpose in life, satisfying our need for meaning?

Surely, there is more to life than struggling to survive. There is more to life than accumulating assets and making things secure. And there is more to life than fame and fortune. There is more to life than pleasure and freedom and food and friends and even physical health. There is self-actualization. There is more.

Self-actualizing is a process of being authentic and living genuinely. It is discovering your real self, not the ego or the mistaken beliefs you may have had, but a Higher Self, and letting that "actualize."

Self-actualizing people are described as having positive self-perception, acceptance of self and others, a relaxed openness to life, full-functioning personal abilities, self-confidence, a sense of humor without hostility, and "peak" experiences, almost mystical experiences of beauty, goodness, and love. They have a life that values unity, richness, beauty, effortlessness, playfulness, honesty, and self-sufficiency.

Sounds good to me. Put me down for that.

MY TAKE? WE HAVE A NEED TO BE WELL OR WHOLE

When we feel like having something to eat, and it has nothing to do with our nutrient needs, we need to ask ourselves "What's missing?"

We have needs: physical, mental, and spiritual. As grown-ups, we need to take responsibility to see that we satisfy them. If you solved your weight problem, but ignored this issue, you may still have the emptiness, or you may still be trying to fill it with another wrong thing. We need to get this right. How? Answer this:

What comes first in your life? Your kids? Your spouse? Your job? Yourself?

Earlier, I had said that for us to work with clients, weight control and health had to be their number one priority. It had to come first, before anything else. That conflicted with some mental health and religious people who said that idea was off-center and unhealthy. They had differing ideas of what should be at the center of your life, the thing that comes first.

Let me suggest something. Make real health your number one priority. Everything else will fall into place. Make *wholeness*— body, mind, and spirit— number one. They are the same thing. The word "health" comes from "heal," which means to "make whole." To be whole means to have nothing missing, to be complete, rather than missing a piece.

To be whole means to have all your needs met: the physical, security, social, family, ego, and even the self-actualization needs— all your needs, body, mind, and spirit. To be whole has also meant union, or re-union, with whatever it is that we are all made of, that one thing at our center, the energy that forms all matter, the thought that is the cause of all things, that forms us all and everything in our existence— to be one with it, "right with God" in the language of the religious.

Decide that being *whole* is the number one issue in your life. Make it the most important thing, so that you'll do nothing that interferes with it, and you'll work to do whatever makes it happen. Measure every decision and action you make against this test: does it help or hurt your effort to become whole, body, mind, and spirit? Make it so that being whole and healthy comes first in your life. With that, all your needs will be met.

CHAPTER 15

Ready, Set, Go!
Save Yourself First.

Are you ready to solve the obesity problem? If you are, start with yourself.

You can start today. If you want to work with a therapist, and you are close to one of my associated therapists, you can call and make an appointment. Go to my website, **www.theandersonmethod.com** and check.

If you want to try it on your own, I heartily encourage you. After all, therapists only *help* people, they don't do the work or make the changes. The client is the one who does that.

I, and many others, studied, just as you are doing, tried and failed many times, just as you have done, but we eventually "got it." You can, too. If you want the assistance a therapist and training program can give you, it will always be an option. Coaches and teachers and training programs can be a big help, whether it is sports, business, or some other ability; but it is you who does the work and makes the difference, with or without the assistance. Give it a try.

Today, go to the bookstore, and get a calorie reference. My favorite is *The Calorie Counter* by Annette Natow and Jo-Ann

Heslin, both registered dieticians, who have been putting out this simple but comprehensive source book for years. It lists the calories in generic and brand name foods, and it has a section for chain restaurants, too. It lists only calories, so it is easy to read, without the confusing array of all the other nutrient counts. To get started, all we are interested in is the calories. That's all that matters for weight control purposes.

After you get your calorie book, start keeping track of what you eat, the specific food you eat, and the quantity of it. Keep a notebook, and list everything you eat during the day. Don't try to "diet" or cut back yet. The idea, at first, is to get an idea of where the calories have been coming from when you eat "normally" — to develop a consciousness or awareness of what you've been doing. At the end of the day, sit down and add up the calories in what you ate. Do this for at least a week before you try to make any changes.

It will be work, and it's not a lot of fun, but it is incredibly enlightening. You will be amazed at what you discover. It will be one of the most eye-opening experiences of your life.

If you can get yourself to do this, you will be on your way. If you can't, you probably need the structure of a training program. If you do, don't feel bad. Many great people do.

Keep track of everything you eat while you finish the book, for at least a week, before you make any changes in your eating.

If you are honest, and you get a number every day that reflects an accurate total of the calories you consumed, you will be on the right track and ready to proceed at the end of the week. That means you have to do the work to find out what's in the food you're eating, and how many calories are in it. You'll have to analyze what's in your dishes, and come up with a calorie total. You'll have to go to the recipes and come up with totals and find out what's in the serving you had. You'll have to weigh and measure. It's work, a real pain in the neck, but like I tell my clients, if you do this right, you only need to do it once in your life.

You also need to know your estimated metabolic rate, the number of calories you burn each day, so you can compare that with what you've been eating. We use a simple method that has been used by dieticians for years, not as precise as some other methods, but accurate enough for our purposes. We estimate that you burn, assuming average activity and exercise habits (a half hour per day,) fifteen calories per pound, per day, of your *Ideal Body Weight (IBW)*. So, take your *Ideal Body Weight* (not your current weight or the weight you want to be,) multiply that by fifteen, and you'll have your estimated metabolic rate, the approximate number of calories you burn per day.

Ideal Body Weight is a clinical term, and it has nothing to do with what you think *your* ideal weight is. It is the weight that actuarial scientists have found is the healthiest weight to be, the weight where we have the lowest morbidity and mortality. It is the weight that has been on those charts at the doctors' offices for years, the ones that seemed so hopelessly unrealistic for us. For women, it is one hundred pounds for the first five feet in height, plus five pounds per inch, over five feet. For men, it is 106 pounds for the first five feet in height, plus six pounds per inch over five feet.

Find your IBW, multiply that by fifteen, and you'll get your approximate burn rate. As an example, for a woman five feet, four inches the IBW would be [100 + (4x5=20) =120]; multiply that by fifteen, and get 1,800 calories per day.

Many people, doctors and dieticians included, have misinterpreted and misapplied this method, most often thinking that we burn fifteen calories per day of body weight. They think that a person who weighs three hundred pounds must burn 4,500 calories per day, and that if you want to weigh 150 pounds, you should get into the habit of eating 2,250 calories per day. This is a bad mistake. Many people have been misled by this confusion and have suffered a great deal because of it.

Remember, if you have normal activity habits, your metabolic rate depends on your muscle mass more than any other factor, and that is a function of your height, your frame size, not your weight. The method of determining your estimated metabolic rate based on your IBW is actually a method based on height.

Go out and get a calorie book tonight or tomorrow, and start keeping track of what you eat. Eat normally for the next week. Don't diet or make any changes in what you do just yet. Get an accurate number every day, and compare that with what you burn. Start getting an idea of what happened. Remember, our weight is a result of an energy balance, and weight gain or loss is the result of a *cumulative* imbalance. You will be thunderstruck when you begin to understand the impact that our way of life and our way of eating has been having on our bodies. You will begin to see why the obesity rate has doubled and quadrupled in the last thirty years, since the birth of our "consumer" culture. You will be horrified to imagine where it's going— we seem to be getting worse rather than better, embracing the "good life" of consuming, more and more each year, addicts given up to their addiction.

It needn't continue that way.

When you have finished this book, get a pad of paper, and start re-reading this book. Make notes, as you go, of ideas you want to use. Make lists of the things you want to do, the changes you want to make, the new habits you want to develop, and what you'll do to make it happen.

This book is crammed with information you need, and if you're normal, you've forgotten at least half of it already. Take your time re-reading it, making notes, and formulating your plan.

After a week of eating "normally," begin *undereating* with the weekday/weekend pattern I've described. We target one-third of our burn rate for five weekdays (but never under eight hundred) and at least two-thirds on the weekend days (only two days, your choice.)

On week*days*, we work to hit the target, and on weekends we work to keep it in a range. On week*days*, we are more rigid, and on weekends we are flexible.

On week*ends*, we can eat up to our burn rate, but *never over* the burn rate.

Form a plan of what you'll be doing each day, pulling ideas especially from the chapters on modeling, undereating, and Therapeutic Psychogenics; but first, eat the way you normally eat, for a week, while you keep track of the calories; and begin re-reading this book, making notes, lists, and plans.

While you are doing that, finish the book and consider the possibilities of success on a grander scale than perhaps you had ever considered.

CHAPTER 16

Beating the Obesity Epidemic and Saving the World.

In the beginning of the book, I had reported that the CDC described obesity as an epidemic, with the rate of obesity growing at a rate that parallels infectious diseases. I reported that obesity is the second leading cause of preventable death in the country, second only to smoking. It will probably soon overtake smoking, causing over 300,000 deaths per year, and growing. These are not exaggerations. It is not sensational talk. It is fact.

You have probably sensed that your overeating habits have characteristics that seem similar to an addiction, and you are right.

We are addicted, as individuals and as a culture, to overeating, to overconsuming, and it is one of the toughest addictions to beat. It is killing us, and killing the planet.

And you can save it.

HOW TO SAVE THE WORLD

You have the opportunity to lead a heroic life by doing something that you may have thought was totally selfish.

Whenever we wanted to lose weight and look better, to feel better about our lives and our bodies, it was for selfish reasons.

Here is the chance to do something truly great, perhaps the one thing that needs to be done to save the world, while you are doing the single most important thing just for yourself. What an incredible coincidence.

The world is addicted to consuming, just as we have been, and it has been consuming itself to death.

When you change, and you reject the way you have been acting and thinking, something miraculous will occur. When you truly commit yourself to wholeness and health, and begin undereating, and work each day to improve your life, your most heartfelt dreams will begin to materialize. You will begin to lose weight. You will begin to look better and feel better about yourself. Your health will improve, your clothes will feel better, and look better, but something more important will happen.

Your change will change something greater than you.

Others will see you and hear what you say. When you start acting and talking in a way that reflects a commitment to healthy living, healthy eating, and healthy thinking, others will be affected. You will model for them, and you will lead them. You don't even need to try. It will happen. It has always happened. But now, it will be in a healthy direction, and your world will change. You will be better for it, and the world will be better for it.

YOU ARE THE WORLD

Just as the cells of your skin or your heart are parts of you, you are a part of the world, a cell of that greater being.

When a cell is infected with disease, and it is allowed to grow, the disease grows and spreads, and the whole body can become sick with it, perhaps sick to death.

Healing and wholeness can spread the same way.

When you take control of your little piece, your life, and you commit it to what you want more than anything, to make yourself happy and healthy, not only will you save yourself and your dreams. Something bigger will happen.

You will lose weight and feel better, but you will also generate a wholeness in yourself that will infect others and spread. It can spread everywhere, if you push it. It can overcome the disease, it can overcome the addiction.

Life and wholeness grow.

Disease and sickness, addiction included, do not. They burn themselves out, kill their host and themselves, and result in nothing.

When you make health and wholeness your cause, something great will happen. When, from the moment you wake, your thought, mind, and life are focused on real health, things will get better. It will grow.

To do this, all you need to do now is focus on your own well-being. Imagine yourself at the weight you want to be, feeling better, looking better, smiling, happy. It can happen.

Go to the book store today, and start tracking, and after you finish this book, start re-reading it and make those notes, lists, and plans. You can always opt for working with a therapist if you want to.

You have a better life to live, and it has begun already. It will change your world.

CHAPTER 17

Now what?

When you go to the bookstore, you'll see lots of diets. Diets to lose weight, diets to live longer, diets to be smarter— it's as if what you put in your mouth is the answer to everything. These diets are so concerned about what and what not to eat— avoiding additives, eating organic, or vegetarian— afraid of carbs, or fat, or meat, or butter, or eggs, or coffee. It's as if what goes into your mouth is the most important thing in determining what will happen in your life.

However, long ago, thousands of years before there were such people as cognitive psychologists and Cognitive Behavior Therapy, we were taught that we are not hurt by what we put *into* our mouths, but by what comes *out*— our words, the thoughts we think.

The religions of the times, like the popular culture of today, seemed to be focused on what to eat, and what not to eat, and when— as if *that* was the way to a blessed life. Some questioned the high priests of the times, whom we could liken to the media moguls and marketplace gurus of today, saying we were hurt not so much by eating the wrong things as *thinking* the wrong things.

While we certainly have a desperate need to be conscious of what we are eating, our food diet, it is really more important to pay attention to our *mental* diet, the thoughts we feed our mind— the thoughts and the way of thinking that we engage in every day, all day long.

What's your mental diet like?

What TV do you watch? What do you read? Who do you listen to? What are your hobbies?

If your diet is a steady stream of sensational TV "news," cynical situation "comedies," and "reality" shows, and toxic "friends" with their complaints and forecasts of doom and gloom, your mental diet is the equivalent of a lethal dose of cyanide. Does your mental diet include shock radio, negative internet or video game stuff, tabloid trash, or stories of the rich and infamous?

Stop it.

We need to pay attention to our mental diet and work to put healthy thinking through our minds from here on in, just as we must work, the rest of our lives, to have healthy eating and activity habits. Because we live in the middle of a sick world with a constant barrage of unhealthy messages, we will have to be very intentional about it.

I've talked a lot about managing our self-talk, but we need to pay attention and change what we take in from the world *around* us, too. It's just as important. We can poison ourselves with our own words if we engage in toxic self-talk, but if we indulge in our popular culture, without resisting or altering it, our mind will become a dumping ground for all that's wrong with our world. It's bad news.

We need to work, every day, to intentionally feed our mind the ideas that will promote our well-being, not drain it. We need to plan and carry out plans to feed our mind a diet of ideas and thinking that will lift our spirit, promote our healthiest visions, and reveal the best that we have in us. We need to stop putting our mind on the road to ruin and put it on the path to our highest potentials.

After clients complete the initial training in my method, one of their first post-training homework assignments is to visit the bookstore again and get familiar with the self-help, inspirational, recovery or psychology sections, or whatever they call the section that has those kinds of books.

There is a wonderful world of ideas and thinkers waiting for you to discover and embrace them. As you make your way, some will be great, and others may not be, but you will begin a lifetime task of building your knowledge and wisdom, and more importantly, your well-being. It will take you the rest of your life, but that's a good thing. The alternative is to spend the rest of your life taking in the trash.

We need to plan our days and activities to put us in contact with healthy people with healthy thoughts. You may need to change friends or the gathering places you attend. You may even need to change jobs and who you're living with. Your life, or the quality of your life, which is the same thing, depends on it.

When you do this, your life will change. Your world will change. You will become one of the voices that lift others and lights their way. You don't even have to try to do this. It will just happen as a result of your improving your own life.

It has already begun.

Keep reading.

ACKNOWLEDGEMENTS

I owe a great debt to many people, a few who I will name, and many who I will not. Rules of confidentiality, and considerations of reason and privacy, limit me in that regard. I hope that I will be able to return all that I have received and more, through their generosity and grace.

Deeply-felt thanks go to Deborah Greenleaf for her constant encouragement and for her willingness to read everything I have written and provide her invaluable feedback. Her generous spirit is an inspiration, and her relation a divine gift.

Thanks go to all my clients who have worked hard to develop themselves and the success they desire. They have worked so hard to complete the tasks I led them to, and they've blessed me with the opportunity to witness the success it brought. My thanks go to them for using what I could give them and encouraging me to believe in the value of my work. To them, I wish continued progress as we take what we have received and keep working.

Over the years, there are many who have given me so much and who deserve so much in return, and I acknowledge here a few: My family, especially my mother and father, Chris Anderson and my children, Amber and Lincoln; and also Tom Henson, George and Carol Belcher, Mark Lupo, Fred Bloom, Linda Carson, Waldo Proffitt, and so many more I hope to richly reward for their belief and support. I hope to earn it, and I pray that my success in that regard comes more surely and quickly than my success with my weight and other mundane responsibilities. Many thanks to you all.

ABOUT THE AUTHOR

W illiam Anderson is a Licensed Mental Health Counselor residing in Florida. He is a graduate of the University of Massachusetts, Amherst (B.S.), and the University of South Florida Graduate School of Education, Tampa (M.A.). He conducts a private psychotherapy practice in Sarasota, Florida, and is currently training other therapists to provide The Anderson Method in their own practices. He serves Sarasota's community mental health efforts as a clinical volunteer at Genesis Health Center for the uninsured and medically indigent, and is an avid fisherman, cook, and lifelong student.

To learn more about The Anderson Method program of therapy, prospective clients and therapists should visit **www. theandersonmethod.com**.